MOTIVATIONAL INTERVIEWING IN MEDICAL REHABILITATION

ACADEMY OF REHABILITATION PSYCHOLOGY SERIES

Series Editors

Lisa A. Brennar, Editor-in-Chief
Bruce Caplan
Timothy Elliott
Janet Farmer
Robert Frank
Barry Nierenberg
George Prigatano
Daniel Rohe
Stephen T. Wegener

Volumes in the Series

Ethics Field Guide: Applications in Rehabilitation Psychology
Thomas R. Kerkhoff and Stephanie L. Hanson

The Social Psychology of Disability
Dana S. Dunn

Disability-Affirmative Therapy: A Case Formulation Template for Clients with
Disabilities
Rhoda Olkin

Validity Assessment in Rehabilitation Psychology and Settings
Dominic A. Carone and Shane S. Bush

Suicide Prevention after Neurodisability: An Evidence-Informed Approach
Grahame K. Simpson and Lisa A. Brenner

Understanding the Experience of Disability: Perspectives from Social and
Rehabilitation
Psychology
Dana S. Dunn

Disability as Diversity: Developing Cultural Competence
Erin E. Andrews

Motivational Interviewing in Medical Rehabilitation

IMPROVING PATIENT ENGAGEMENT AND TEAM FUNCTION

Edited by Nicole Schechter, Connie Jacocks, Lester Butt, and Stephen T. Wegener

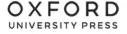

OXFORD
UNIVERSITY PRESS

OXFORD
UNIVERSITY PRESS

Oxford University Press is a department of the University of Oxford. It furthers
the University's objective of excellence in research, scholarship, and education
by publishing worldwide. Oxford is a registered trade mark of Oxford University
Press in the UK and certain other countries.

Published in the United States of America by Oxford University Press
198 Madison Avenue, New York, NY 10016, United States of America.

© Oxford University Press 2024

CIP data is on file at the Library of Congress
ISBN 978–0–19–774826–8

DOI: 10.1093/oso/9780197748268.001.0001

Printed by Marquis Book Printing, Canada

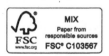

The editors dedicate this work to the rehabilitation community—
our colleagues and the people we serve.

Contents

Foreword

What does motivational interviewing (MI) have to do with rehabilitation or more generally with healthcare? After all, Steve Rollnick and I originally developed it in the 1980s to help people reduce harmful alcohol use. What we didn't appreciate at the time was how ambivalence about change is an important issue in so many different fields and professions. Beyond addictions, MI quickly found a home in healthcare, especially in managing long-term medical conditions like diabetes where the patient's active involvement in their health is a major factor determining their future wellness and quality of life. MI also began being used in correctional systems to help offenders choose a more pro-social life path and in education to promote active student engagement in their own learning. Applications of MI emerged in preventive dentistry, mental health counseling, nutrition and fitness, coaching, social work, public health, leadership, and management. As it turns out, ambivalence is human nature (Miller, 2021).

It makes sense, then, that MI is also applicable in physical and cognitive rehabilitation to help people take an active role in their own recovery. In a way, your job as a rehabilitation professional is to ask and encourage people to do things that are necessary for recovery and that they might not want to do. That's not the whole story, actually, because there is usually a part of the patient that does want to have better functioning and life quality. That part of patients is your primary ally in rehabilitation. No one knows more about your patients than they do themselves, and if you're asking them to do something difficult, then you need their own wisdom and expertise as well as your own. MI is a blending of expertise—yours and theirs—to discover how best to help them move forward toward health and wellness.

Those of us who choose helping professions usually want to help, to make a difference for the better in the lives of people we serve. How best to do that? We helpers often have a fixing reflex, a tendency to try to repair the person—to educate, coach, and cajole them into changing. Sometimes healthcare practitioners do know how to fix certain problems: mend a broken bone, recognize and treat an infection, or alleviate pain. Nevertheless, the patient still has a vital role in such treatment—to rest and elevate, take the medication, do the exercises. Ask yourself, "Is this something that I can fix myself?" If so, fix it. What we cannot do for patients is to make changes in their behavior and lifestyle, much as we might wish to do so. When such change is what's needed, we need to activate the patient's own motivations and resources.

That's what Steve Rollnick and I developed MI to do. He and I could tell our patients "You have to stop drinking," but it wasn't true. We could recite reasons why we thought change would be a good idea, but usually patients aren't all that interested in why we hope they will change. What matters in rehabilitation is why they might choose to change, improve, exercise, eat better, or get stronger. We could explain how change could be accomplished, but it is the patient who ultimately decides whether and how to do it. MI is about evoking—literally calling forth—from people their own motivations for and ideas about positive change. If you do it well, they may not think that you did much for them because they did it themselves.

Does it work? There have now been more than 2,000 controlled clinical trials involving MI, most often used in combination with other effective treatments. I have been saying lately that MI is a way of doing what else you do; it is how and who you are in relationship with your patients. Core skills of MI such as empathic listening, affirming, and evoking change talk are more generally characteristics of effective helpers, the "bedside manner" of better healers (Miller & Moyers, 2021). But how do you actually do these things? What does it look like in practice? Many helpers believe that they are already good listeners and have gifts of empathy and encouragement. What we have contributed in MI research is clearer knowledge about exactly how to strengthen your skills and improve your practice in these areas. These are measurable, learnable skills that make a real difference in your patients' outcomes above and beyond the technical procedures of practice.

I am grateful to the editors and contributors of *Motivational Interviewing in Medical Rehabilitation* for making this evidence-based method more accessible to you as practitioners who accompany patients on the journey to recovery. Learning about MI is just a beginning. As in sports and music, it is intentional practice that makes a difference in your skillfulness, perhaps with the assistance of a coach to guide your early learning. May you discover what many other learners have found, that practicing MI can make your work more enjoyable, lift a burden from your shoulders, yield fairly rapid changes in how patients respond to you, and improve their outcomes.

William R. Miller, Ph.D.
Emeritus Distinguished Professor of Psychology and Psychiatry
The University of New Mexico

References

Miller, W. R. (2021). *On second thought: How ambivalence shapes your life*. Guilford Publications.
Miller, W. R., & Moyers, T. B. (2021). *Effective psychotherapists*. Guilford Publications.

Contributors

Asma Ali, PsyD, ABPP-RP
Centered Peak Behavioral Health &
Wellness

**Kathleen T. Bechtold, PhD,
ABPP-RP, CN**
Johns Hopkins University School of
Medicine

Charles H. Bombardier, PhD, ABPP-RP
University of Washington

Lester Butt, PhD, ABPP-RP
Craig Hospital

Amanda Choflet, DNP, RN
Northeastern University

Kelly Daley, PT, MBA
Johns Hopkins University School of
Medicine

Joe Fangman, MS, PT
Craig Hospital

Ruth Grenoble, LCSW, CCM
Craig Hospital

Allie Hamilton, PT, DPT
Craig Hospital

Sarah Horan, MS, OTR/L
Craig Hospital

Connie Jacocks, PhD, ABPP-CN
Vista Neuropsychology

Linda Ehrlich-Jones, RN, PhD
Shirley Ryan Ability Lab &
Northwestern University Feinberg
School of Medicine

Annette Lavezza, OTR/L
Johns Hopkins University School of
Medicine

Danbi Lee, PhD, OTD, OTR/L
University of Washington

Emily Markley, PsyD
Ardent Grove Foundation

William R. Miller, PhD
University of New Mexico

Jennifer Rikard, PhD
San Diego State University

Nicole Schechter, PsyD, ABPP-RP
Johns Hopkins University School of
Medicine

**Maureen Gecht-Silver, OTD,
MPH, OTR/L**
University of Illinois Chicago

Laura Torres, LCSW-C
Johns Hopkins Health System

**Kristen Mascareñas Wendling, MA,
CCC-SLP**
Craig Hospital

Stephen T. Wegener, PhD, ABPP-RP
Johns Hopkins University School of
Medicine

Katherine S. Wright, PhD
University of Washington

Introduction and Acknowledgments

REHABILITATION AND THE management of chronic health conditions require patients to be proactive and engaged in their healthcare. This need for active partnership between patients and rehabilitation professionals takes place in an evolving healthcare environment. Specifically, this calls for patient-centered care with a greater focus on patient satisfaction and improved outcomes. Clinicians need strategies and tools to build trusting therapeutic alliance, support goal-setting, and promote behavior change that engage patients as partners in care and make patient-centered care a reality.

Motivational interviewing (MI) is an evidence-based approach that has been shown to change behaviors and increase engagement in many patient populations. The foundational concepts and skills of MI emphasize building a collaborative partnership between the clinician and patient (and family) in which the individual's autonomy is respected and their personal goals are clarified and pursued. This empowers individuals toward goal attainment and independence. MI spirit and skills are an ideal fit with the ethos and needs of the rehabilitation community.

The goals of this book are to (1) provide rehabilitation professionals with the foundations of MI, (2) describe how this approach can be applied by a range of rehabilitation disciplines to address common barriers to rehabilitation engagement, and (3) provide guidance for those interested in implementing MI training in rehabilitation settings. Chapters are authored by rehabilitation experts from the many disciplines found on the interdisciplinary or transdisciplinary rehabilitation team. The

Introduction and Acknowledgments In: *Motivational Interviewing in Medical Rehabilitation.* Edited by: Nicole Schechter, Connie Jacocks, Lester Butt, and Stephen T. Wegener, Oxford University Press. © Oxford University Press 2024.
DOI: 10.1093/oso/9780197748268.003.0001

author group is comprised of physical therapists, physiatrists, occupational therapists, psychologists, speech and language pathologists, social workers, and nurses.

The reader interested in building foundational MI skills would do well to begin with the Section I chapters before going on to subsequent chapters, which describe the application of MI to specific clinical situations. Those with a foundation in MI may choose to skip the Section I chapters and focus on the chapters describing the application of MI in specific situations.

A unique dimension of this book is the interplay with the website www.rehabeng age.org. At this website there are video presentations on MI spirit and skills as well as video demonstrations by rehabilitation professionals using these skills in a variety of clinical situations. At various points in this volume the reader is referred to the website for video presentation of materials covered in the text. This provides the reader with the opportunity to see the MI spirit and skills in action. While the book is intended for practicing rehabilitation clinicians, educators preparing students for careers in rehabilitation will find several tools to assist them in their efforts, including recommended readings and learner reflection/discussion questions.

This book should be viewed in the evolving context of MI knowledge, terminology and practice. The recent publication—*Motivational interviewing: Helping people change and grow, 4th Edition* (Miller and Rollnick, 2023)—emphasizes the beautiful simplicity of MI, while appreciating the complexity of human relationships. We endeavored to incorporate the new terminology that is introduced in the 4th Edition, while keeping a focus on basic principles to make MI accessible for the rehabilitation community. The 4th Edition, and our efforts, reflect the values of the MI community—partnership and openness to positive change.

The making of this book would not have been possible without this dedicated team of interdisciplinary authors. Thank you for your hard work for this book and the hard work you do every day to support the rehabilitation community.

The editors would like to acknowledge those who supported, inspired, and made this possible:

- Nicole Schechter would like to thank her family—Howie, Corinne, Sloane, Dara, Ron, and Noah—for the love and laughs.
- Lester Butt wishes to acknowledge his two families: Candice, Evan, and Grahm and his Craig Hospital family.
- Connie Jacocks would like to acknowledge her family—Marc, Charlie, and Myra—for their support and encouragement and colleagues past and present who have been so generous with their time in providing guidance and mentorship.

- Stephen T. Wegener would like to thank Lisa for sharing her expertise in MI and living the MI spirit. Because of her—this book, our family and my life are the better.
- All of us would like to thank Tricia Kirkhart for her passion and dedication that make this work possible.

Finally, to those reading, we appreciate your dedication to improving care in rehabilitation. We hope the spirit and skills covered in this book will be as helpful in your work as they are in ours.

Nicole Schechter
Connie Jacocks
Lester Butt
Stephen T. Wegener

Reference

Miller, W. R., & Rollnick, S. (2023). *Motivational interviewing: Helping people change and grow.* Guilford Publications.

SECTION I

Foundations

1 Motivational Interviewing

PHILOSOPHICAL UNDERPINNINGS AND SPIRIT

Lester Butt and Stephen T. Wegener

Introduction

This chapter presents the philosophical underpinnings of motivational inter-viewing (MI) and the values and spirit that arise from these philosophies. This chapter attempts to summarize and place in the rehabilitation context the key foundations, values, and spirit of MI. For more detailed and masterful presenta-tion, we recommend Miller and Rollnick's book (2023). You can also learn more at https://www.rehabengage.org/, a resource constructed by the book's editors (Schechter et al., 2021). Briefly stated, MI is not a set of techniques but a way of being with patients, families, and team members. It is an evidence based way of to promote change and growth. The spirit and values of MI are reflected in the current definition:

> "MI is a particular way of talking with people about change and growth to strengthen their own motivation and commitment." (Miller & Rollnick, 2023, p. 3)

Lester Butt and Stephen T. Wegener, *Motivational Interviewing* In: *Motivational Interviewing in Medical Rehabilitation.* Edited by: Nicole Schechter, Connie Jacocks, Lester Butt, and Stephen T. Wegener, Oxford University Press.
© Oxford University Press 2024. DOI: 10.1093/oso/9780197748268.003.0002

Before we explore MI further, let's look at a common situation we encounter in the rehabilitation team meeting:

The team is meeting about a person with spinal cord injury who has been on the unit for some time. The team is dealing with, and talking about, a patient who has not grasped a main tenet of rehabilitation—that the patient needs to be an active participant in their care. The individual is reluctant to go to therapy, saying "If I rest, I will get better." He is reluctant to participate in self-care, cathing, and skin checks and would like to eat in his room rather than participate in any group interaction. When asked to participate, he is often irritable and angry. The team members are discussing the situation and making comments:

This person isn't using our program.... It is frustrating he doesn't do more... he has so much potential. ...We need to set a strict behavioral plan and let him know what our rules are.... Maybe we need to just give him more time to get on board.... I think we need to educate him how if he doesn't do his self-cares he will have a lot of problems and can't go home and may need to go to a nursing home.... I think he's depressed and we need to do a diagnostic interview and perhaps start meds.... If he just listened to us, then he would do better and would see progress.

As you read through this chapter, reflect on how the values and spirit are, or are not, reflected in these comments. We will revisit the team and see how this conversation might be different if infused with MI values and spirit. In this next section we explore how MI values and spirit are a seamless fit for the context and challenges faced in rehabilitation.

MI and Rehabilitation

Rehabilitation professionals reading this chapter will find themselves recognizing, and being familiar with, the values and spirit of MI. This should not be surprising as many of the values are shared. Indeed, one of the inspirations for the authors in putting together this book was that the shared values and spirit of MI would draw rehabilitation professionals into using these tasks and skills to make these mutual foundations fully present in their work. Rehabilitation values include the following: accepting that different patients have different levels of ability and that individuals have retained strengths; patient choices are to be respected; patients/families bear physical, psychological, and social burdens; identifying the patient's goals and using those to guide treatment planning is key; the patient and family are at the center of the team; and collaboration is needed to optimize function. These rehabilitation values are mirrored in the MI spirit of acceptance, marked by respect for autonomy, affirming strengths, and empathy; showing compassion for the individual's situation and struggle; empowering and seeking to understand the individual's wisdom, motivations, and priorities; and developing a partnership with the patient/ family to achieve engagement and goals.

Further, in addition to guiding our interactions with patients and families, the values and spirit can be the foundation for our interactions with team members. Our colleagues also deserve respect for their autonomy and strengths; compassion for the multiple burdens they bear; understanding of their beliefs, motivations, and goals; and developed partnerships to serve their patients and one another. Please see Chapter 2 for a deeper dive into how MI can be used in rehabilitation contexts. Let's now examine some key factors that can help us reify and realize these values.

Communication Principles and Constructive Conversations

In the healing arts, we have several main tools that have been available since ancient times—the herb, the knife, and the word. We have made life-changing advances in medication and surgery. One unintended consequence of these advances was a loss of value in the patient–professional relationship and the power of language in healing. Of course, this was never totally lost. The paradigm shift of the biopsychosocial model in the 1980s (Engel, 1977), the growth of self-management and other cognitive and behavioral approaches in the 1990s, and the focus of the Institute of Medicine (IOM) on patient-centered care since 2000 (IOM, 2001) all renewed interest in the healing relationship and the language that facilitates constructive growth.

In this section we will first reflect on communication styles and interpersonal responses that arise in healthcare interactions. In the next section we turn to the values and spirit of MI that build a trusting therapeutic alliance and support productive goal-setting and treatment interactions.

COMMUNICATION STYLES

The spirit of MI is reflected in our style of communication. Communication between healthcare professionals and patients is usually marked by the professional being the in-charge expert, responsible for fixing the problem, and encouraging the person to engage and/or change. In contrast, an MI-consistent conversation is marked by the professional having expertise to offer and being patient-focused and collaborative and eliciting the individual's own goals and motivations for change. These two styles are outlined in Table 1.1. Most of us recognize the value of the MI style. However, when

TABLE 1.1

MI Spirit and Communication Style

Traditional fixer style	MI style
• Goal-oriented	• Patient-oriented
• Expert role	• Collaborative
• Focus on action	• Focus on motivation
• Direct persuasion	• Explore ambivalence
• Give reasons to change	• Elicit reasons to change
• Give warnings	• Elicit concerns
• Clinician talks more	• Clinician listens more

Note: MI = motivational interviewing.

faced with challenging patients and the pressure of shortened lengths of stay and/ or limited encounters, we may revert to more traditional, overlearned approaches.

Looking more closely at communication patterns, we see key elements that come together to produce three communication styles. These styles are depicted in Figure 1.1. The three elements that characterize conversations can be divided into *informing* (telling, educating), *asking questions*, and *listening*. The different emphasis of each of these different elements gives rise to markedly different ways of communicating.

In the *directing* style there exists a high level of informing, limited asking, and limited listening. Words associated with this style are *manage*, *in charge*, and *tell*. Traditional healthcare provider–patient conversations are often marked by this style. We have expertise to offer, there is a person presenting with a problem, and

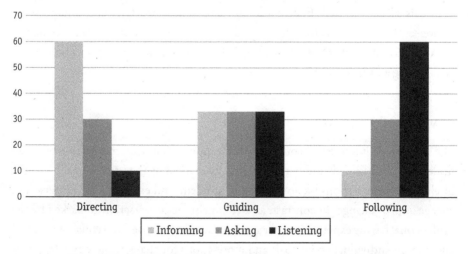

FIGURE 1.1 Three Communication Styles

we want to help them solve it. For many of us, this is a comfortable style and at times a productive and efficient way to interact. On the other end of the spectrum, there is the *following* style. This style is marked by a lot of listening, some questioning, and limited informing. Words associated with this style are *observe*, *permit*, and *go along with*. We often see this style in traditional counseling interactions where the provider is helping a client make a decision such as choosing a major in college. Herein there is no overarching right choice, and the provider has no investment in the choice or subsequent behavior. The third style is *guiding*. This style is marked by a balance of asking, listening, and informing. Words associated with this style are *shepherd*, *collaborate*, and *awaken*. This is the style we often see in effective teachers who inquire as to what the student already knows and what they would like to learn and who provide information in a manner that meets the student at their own level.

There is no one right style. Different situations call for different styles. For example, in various healthcare settings different styles may be more appropriate and effective. The directing style may be useful and effective in the emergency department, where the focus is on action and where limited patient engagement is required. The following style may be useful in the context of palliative care, where patient preferences are paramount and asking and listening are essential and necessary. We believe that rehabilitation calls for a guiding style with an equal balance of asking, listening, and informing, thereby leading to patient engagement and improved outcomes. This style is most effective in situations such as rehabilitation, chronic disease care, and primary care where patient/family engagement is essential to achieving optimal outcomes and where patient preferences and resources are diverse. As we look at some key interpersonal factors in communication, we will see how the guiding style helps us avoid some traps and pitfalls that can undermine the therapeutic alliance, prevent progress, and reduce patient/provider satisfaction.

In the light of conversational styles, MI can be conceptualized as "refined guiding" in that it involves a purposeful conversation, using balanced conversational elements to elicit the patient's own arguments for change and engagement. If you find yourself doing most of the talking in patient interactions, you need to ask, "Am I truly guiding?"

READER REFLECTION QUESTIONS

Before moving forward, let's bring this closer to home. Take a moment to reflect:

- What is your natural style?
- What is the style that you revert to when in a stressful situation—when tired or working with a difficult patient or team member?
- How can I be more aware when I am using an ineffective style?

INTERPERSONAL FACTORS IN COMMUNICATION

Conversations take place between two or more individuals. It is helpful to keep in mind several natural human responses that emerge as we engage in these conversations—be they patient–professional or another interpersonal context. Here, we are going to highlight two responses that are at the heart of MI—ambivalence and the drive to provide our solutions to problems as they are presented to us.

Individuals considering change, called to adapt to a new situation or develop new skills—all part of the rehabilitation process—are often ambivalent. *Ambivalence* is having mixed or conflicting feelings/thoughts about a particular decision or behavior. This is a normal and universal process. We encounter this when we, or those around us, consider developing a new health habit—stopping smoking, starting to exercise, becoming a vegetarian, or starting a new medication. It is seen in other situations—"Should we move or remodel" or "Should I stay in this relationship or break up." Ambivalence is demonstrated within all of us; none of us are immune. This concept is reflected in the transtheoretical model (TTM) of Prochaska and DiClemente (1992). The TTM and the supporting data indicate that individuals move through a series of five stages—precontemplation, contemplation, preparation, action, maintenance—as they adopt healthy behaviors or cease unhealthy ones. In this process individuals' thoughts are often marked by ambivalence that must be addressed to help move through the stages to action and maintenance in service of constructive change.

Ambivalence is reflected in the language we and those around us use—"I would like to go to therapy but . . ." or "On the one hand, getting out would be nice, but, on the other hand, people will look at me different." The "yes, but . . ." we hear as clinicians working with patients or families is a clear indicator of ambivalence. Once again, ambivalence is not pathological; it is natural. Resolving ambivalence and moving from *sustain talk*, where the individual is stuck, to *commitment talk*, which leads to action, is a core goal of MI.

Consider what often happens when a healthcare professional encounters this ambivalence when working with a patient. As experts, we know the actions and behaviors that will contribute to health and optimal function and what negative consequences may occur if these actions are not taken. Further, as healers, we want to help people, we want the best for them, and we want to be successful in our work. These factors all lead to the desire to have patients do the "right thing." Of course, this is not just true for patients; it permeates all interactions where we have knowledge to share, care deeply, and want the best for the person. Think of parents with teenagers: They want them to do the "right thing"—be safe, be successful. This leads the clinician, or the parent, to educate, direct, convince, or encourage the person in the direction they believe is best. In MI this is known as the *fixing reflex*, the natural tendency to want to put folks on the right path.

Now let's consider what happens when a person with ambivalence encounters someone who is trying to help and is driven by the fixing reflex. When the clinician takes the positive, pro-health, "let's do it" side of the ambivalent argument, the natural reaction of the patient is to voice the other side.

> CLINICIAN: "Going to therapy would be good for you. You will get stronger, be able to do more for yourself, and get home sooner."
>
> PATIENT: "Yes, but I am really tired because I didn't sleep, and all the people will look at me, and I can't do things easily like before."

Avoiding the fixing reflex and developing an approach infused with MI spirit and skills helps address the ambivalence and avoids pushback, oppositional behavior, and continued avoidance. It has the added benefit of reducing clinician frustration and moving the patient more quickly to action if we avoid the detour of having to address the "yes, but . . ." Later in this book we will present the skills to address ambivalence rather than engaging the fixing reflex. For now, it is helpful to remember that MI is less like bulldozing and more like gardening. It can take time to elicit patient engagement and create sustained health behaviors, but in the long term, the benefits are clearly evident.

READER REFLECTION QUESTIONS

Before moving forward, take a moment to reflect:

- Think of some examples of ambivalence you have encountered in your own life. What was your response when someone tried to persuade you in one direction?
- When patient resistance occurs to your fixing reflex, what is your typical internal and external reaction?
- How can you be more aware when you are caught up in the fixing reflex?

MI Spirit

PHILOSOPHICAL FOUNDATIONS

Our collective multidisciplinary goal as rehabilitation professionals is the enhancement of our clients' quality of life. We enter the field of rehabilitation with the commitment to abet this process and allow our clients and their families to transition to a different life chapter, replete with the requisite skills, safety, heightened confidence, and dignity. This intention occurs irrespective of the nature of the disability or the setting in which our services are provided. Our collective multidisciplinary goal is the highest-achievable-quality outcomes.

The rehabilitation literature is replete with attempts to appreciate the complicated calculus that yields successful outcomes. Early writings spoke to antecedent variables that were believed to be correlated with positive outcomes. As a result, studies explored the relationship between patient-based variables, specifically premorbid psychological variables and their relationship to rehabilitative outcomes.

However, this model proved insufficient in the attempt to more fully understand critical factors that led to positive outcomes. Clinicians and researchers started to envision outcomes predicated on a far broader model. For example, Beatrice Wright (1960), one of the iconic figures in the development of the field of rehabilitation psychology, held that patient active participation in decision-making and establishment of treatment goals and associated interventions were pivotal for maximizing involvement. This stance obviously spoke to the necessity of a collaborative client–professional relationship. Trieschmann (1980) broadly conceptualized rehabilitation as a behavior change process that involved organic factors (age, severity of disability, medical complications, congenital anomalies, strength, endurance), person variables (repertoire of habits, personality style, types of rewards, internal vs. external locus of control, method of coping with stress, self-image, creativity), and environmental variables (hospital milieu, stigma value of disability, family/interpersonal support, financial security, social milieu, urban vs. rural residence, access to medical attention and equipment repair, access to educational/recreation/avocational pursuits, socioeconomic status, architectural barriers and transportation availability, legislation, cultural/ethnic influences).

Far more recently, the areas of motivation, self-efficacy, and outcome expectancies have been discussed as focal points for augmenting positive involvement and outcomes (Lequerica & Kortte, 2010). Many of these contemporary models have involved process variables that were previously not explored. Specifically, for our purposes, one of these process variables involves the specific style/mode of provider–client interaction that is directly associated with desired rehabilitative results. This is not to imply that your client's prior psychosocial history, inclusive of how change/trauma was previously managed, substance abuse issues, family support/networks, nature/extent of disability, etc., is not important. Indeed, these are factors that assuredly impact your client's rehabilitative path. But there are additional crucial supplemental factors that occur within the rehabilitation professional's sphere that have important impacts on outcomes. For example, how you interact with your patients/

families is a determinant of their engagement, participation, and willingness to change. In other words, your interpersonal style is a highly important determinant in your client's success to meet the innumerable demands of rehabilitation.

A very early study that corroborated this stance was conducted by Schontz and Fink (1957). These authors believed that "communicative rapport" between patients and their occupational therapists and physical therapists was an extremely important factor that heightened participation in intensive rehabilitation. As referenced above, in 2001, the IOM issued a report called *Crossing the Quality Chasm*. In this document the IOM challenged the American healthcare system to improve care across several sectors, one of which was labeled *patient-centeredness*. Patient-centered care was enlarged far beyond the acute medical needs of a person to a more holistic model. Patient-centered care included empowering patients to become more active participants in their care, where patient and their providers are accountable for favorable outcomes. Strategies to empower patients included, but were not limited to, the utilization of clinical strategies that augment patient engagement.

This process of engagement is at the core of MI. Within the MI model, the provider is an expert in the rehabilitation process predicated upon their training and experience. Likewise, the client is viewed as an expert on themselves. It is this synergy of provider and client interaction that can fuel participation and continued motivation toward functional independence and accommodation to a disability.

What are the specifics of this constructive provider–client interaction? How do we as providers conceptualize how best to interact with our clients and families? Understanding the basic underpinnings and tenets of MI can begin to answer these important questions prior to discussion of specific MI skills/techniques. Again, Miller and Rollnick (2023, p. 3) define MI as a "particular way of talking with people about change and growth to strengthen their own motivation and commitment." Given this definition, it is apparent how this model of engagement includes pertinent rehabilitative issues: how to assist constructive change as well as how to heighten active involvement and participation of our clients and their families. As such, MI provides a meaningful guide as to how we, as rehabilitation providers, can better serve our clients.

Central to MI is a set of specific skills/techniques—open-ended questions, affirmations, reflective listening, and summary (OARS)—that will be explored in detail in a later Chapter 3. In the early developmental stages of MI, Miller and Rollnick held that these skills formed the essence of their paradigm. However, they soon found these basic skills in isolation to be wanting. Techniques utilized without a necessary MI spirit could result in MI being viewed as a "cynical trick" or a form of "manipulation" (Miller & Rollnick, 2013). They held that the MI spirit is a necessary and essential component that brings both the provider's "mind-set and heart-set"

(Rollnick & Miller, 1995) to their interaction with their clients. They utilize the metaphor of a song to describe the relationship between the MI skills and spirit (Miller & Rollnick, 2002). The song's lyrics represent OARS, the techniques and skills that are essential to operationalize MI. However, the MI spirit is represented by the melody that determines the mood. It is the melody that sets the tone for our client encounters. This spirit is a set of beliefs about human beings often labeled *habits of the heart* that allow us to enter a relationship that creates a collaborative partnership with our clients. The MI spirit, the manner and style of interacting with our clients, is predicated upon a specific vision of human nature, how change occurs, and the clinician's role in facilitating this change.

ACCEPTANCE

Acceptance is not to imply unconditional approval of all our rehabilitation client's behaviors. Indeed, as clinicians, there are specific instances wherein we are called on to oppose/report deleterious behaviors. Those incidents notwithstanding, acceptance has its basic premise deeply embedded within the philosophy of Carl Rogers' client-centered therapy. With the Rogerian model as a backdrop/foundation, Miller and Rollnick (2013, 2023) hold that there are four basic aspects that capture the concept of acceptance.

Absolute Worth

This implies not only the value of every individual with whom we are therapeutically involved but also the belief in the person's innate ability to constructively change. Rogers (1980) referred to this attitude as unconditional positive regard and nonpossessive caring, defined as "an acceptance of this other individual as a separate person, a respect for the other as having worth in his or her own right. It is a basic trust—a belief that this other person is somehow fundamentally trustworthy." Erich Fromm (1956), another noted psychotherapist, discussed "the ability to see a person as he is, to be aware of his unique individuality. Respect means the concern that the other person should grow and unfold as he is. Respect thus implies the absence of exploitation." In addition to the "absence of exploitation," MI calls for us to avoid an authoritative interpersonal stance where the clinician coercively attempts to move the client in a particular direction. Consequently, belief in your client's absolute worth implies the absence of judgment. Rogers (1967) believed that clients who feel unacceptable are "immobilized," with their ability to change thwarted. Conversely, if clients feel accepted, freedom to change is perceived. Lastly, Rogers (1967) believed that if people are provided a genuinely constructive setting, they are driven toward self-actualization, where they naturally choose positive decisions/life directions.

Accurate Empathy

The second ingredient of the Rogerian school of thought involves *accurate empathy*. This is your ability to listen, understand without judgment, and appreciate your client's personal narrative, who they are as a unique individual. It is your ability to see the world through their eyes, understanding their individualized perspective. Rogers (1980) poignantly wrote that accurate empathy is "to sense the client's inner world of private personal meanings as if it were your own, but without ever losing the 'as if' quality." What is a consequence of the rehabilitation practitioner not assuming a stance of accurate empathy? Most probably our clients will feel that their perspective, their frame of reference, is inaccurate, irrelevant, and minimized. This undermines the egalitarian relationship and invitation to change we seek to create.

Autonomy Support

The tenet of autonomy implies respect for your client's self-determination and self-direction. This is the basis of honoring their personhood, their choices. Viktor Frankel (2006), in *Man's Search for Meaning*, written after his internment in a World War II concentration camp, wrote,

> We who lived in concentration camps remember the men who walked through the huts comforting others, giving away their last piece of bread. They may have been few in number, but they offer sufficient proof that everything can be taken from a man but one thing: the last of the human freedoms—to choose one's attitude in any given set of circumstances, to choose one's own way. (p. 44)

The right for each to choose their own way is evident to us working in rehabilitation. We all are aware of those people who choose to believe their lives are over with the onset of physical and/or cognitive impairment compromises. In contrast, we know individuals who choose the path of reconciliation, tolerance, and accommodation to their new lives. We are called to be skillful and accepting guides, respecting and understanding their choices.

Affirmation

The MI spirit is a nonpathological model of human beings: that each of us brings to a situation competencies, strengths, resources, movement toward constructive change, and the will to endure challenges. The rehabilitation provider's intention is to illustrate and reinforce talents and abilities within their clients. This is in direct contrast to typical training wherein our clinical eyes are focused upon deficits, pathology, and weaknesses with a consequent intention to fix our client's problems. Within certain rehabilitation disciplines, it is important to assess and identify areas where remediation is possible. Additionally, it is important to appreciate areas of strength and capabilities. Efforts toward growth and change are not chided if unsuccessful; rather, embracing the MI spirit calls upon the rehabilitation clinician to support the person's efforts, positive direction, and intentions.

Miller and Rollnick (2013) summarize these points eloquently:

> Taken together, these four person-centered conditions convey what we mean by "acceptance." One honors each person's absolute worth and potential as a human being, recognizes and supports the person's irrevocable autonomy to choose his or her own way, seeks through accurate empathy to understand the other's perspective, and affirms the person's strengths and efforts. (p. 19)

It is important to delineate the differences between empathy, altruism, and compassion. *Empathy* can be defined as an emotional experience of another person's feeling, a form of automatic mirroring. *Altruism* is an action that benefits someone else that may or may not be accompanied by empathy or compassion. In distinction, *compassion* involves both an empathic response and altruistic behavior (e.g., an emotional response when perceiving suffering that involves an authentic desire to help). The word *compassion* stems from Latin and Greek roots *pati* and *pathein*, meaning "to suffer," and the Latin root *com*, meaning "with"—that is, the feeling of sorrow or concern for another coupled by the desire to alleviate the suffering (e.g., "I feel for you" + "I understand you" + "I want to help you").

Compassion has a long history within religious tradition, philosophical theory, and psychological writings. For example, consider the following: the Good Samaritan (Christianity), the Golden Rule (Confucius), and the 13 Attributes of Compassion (Judaism). Buddha is believed to have stated, "Loving kindness and compassion is all of our practice." And the Dalai Lama held, "Compassion is a necessity, not a luxury . . . without it, humanity cannot survive" (Dali Lama, n.d.). Additionally, the psychological literature is replete with similar examples of compassionate understanding: "Listening with the 3rd ear" (Reik, 1975), "Vicarious introspection" (Kohut, 1971), "Perceive the internal frame of reference of another with accuracy" (Rogers, 1995), and the "Listening healer" (Jackson, 1992).

It is noteworthy that medical education is seeing a growing emphasis on the inclusion of compassion within the curriculum. For example, Stanford University

Medical School has initiated the Center for Compassion and Altruism Research, and Columbia College of Physicians and Surgeons has an initiative on narrative medicine. In these models, medicine, literature, and the humanities are combined to learn compassion, concern, empathy, understanding, and the essence of human existence in light of illness and disability. Medical students utilize literature and notate in "parallel charts" the more emotional and stressful aspects as experienced by their patients.

All of the above examples illustrate the historical antecedents and the belief in the necessity of compassion. In Friedrich Nietzsche wrote in *Human, All too Human: A Book for Free Spirits*,

> The highest spiritual training of a physician [and rehabilitation professionals] has not yet been reached when he knows and has practical experience in the best and newest methods and understands how to make those rapid deductions from effects to causes for which diagnosticians are famed: he must in addition possess an eloquence that adapts itself to every individual and addresses itself to the heart. (Nietzche, [1878], 2019)

EMPOWERMENT

The MI spirit stands in contrast to the traditional model where the practitioner is the expert, offering diagnosis, interventions, adaptive skills, and experiences to address the client's deficits. The MI spirit believes that the client possesses the requisite internal ability that leads to constructive change. In MI, empowerment "is not primarily giving people something they lack but rather helping them appreciate and use what they already have" (Miller & Rollnick, 2023, p. 7). As a result, the rehabilitation practitioner uses their skills to draw out the internal ability/wisdom/knowledge/solutions from their clients. If this knowledge and solutions emanate from the client, not the provider, there is more belief in their authenticity. Pascal (17th century) wrote in his *Pensées*, "People are generally better persuaded by the reasons which they themselves discovered, than by those which have come into the minds of others" (Pascal, [1670], 2006).Empowerment stems from the principle that your clients are indeed experts in themselves. Our efforts are directed toward client self-exploration and seeking understanding of their abilities and motivations for successful change.

PARTNERSHIP

It is often noted that MI is more like dancing than wrestling, replete with its own natural rhythm. When this concept is operationalized, there is a synchrony between the provider and client, moving in harmony. The successful MI practitioner avoids proscriptive and prescriptive measures. This collaborative relationship is based upon doing "with" and "for," not "to," your client. They are not acted on but are active partners. Within a true provider–client partnership, it is the provider's desire to appreciate the client's worldview and personal narrative, with a clinical eye toward constructive change/accommodation.

It is apparent that within MI there is an emphasis upon both the collaborative relationship and belief in the client's internal resources. This position is underscored by research conducted within the psychotherapy literature. Asay and Lambert (1999) explored both specific factors (technique, manualized treatment approaches, and evidence-based practices) and nonspecific psychotherapeutic practices (client factors, relationship factors and the placebo/hope/expectancy). These authors found that client and relationship factors accounted for 70% of positive outcome variance. This is congruent with the MI model, where belief in the client's abilities coupled with a true partnership were essential components leading toward successful outcomes.

Lastly, a study of what was called "the Roseto effect" is relevant to this discussion. A longitudinal data from 1955 to 1961 was analyzed by Stewart Wolf (1966). The study was the exploration of heart disease, involving Italian immigrants in eastern Pennsylvania who were ostracized by the Welsh and English. Despite this community's smoking, consumption of high-fat diets, working in hazardous slate quarries, and drinking high volumes of wine, it was virtually immune to heart disease, with rates dramatically lower than those for the rest of the United States. This Italian community built its own culture of cooperation replete with a collective civic spirit. The researchers concluded that the Roseto effect on heart disease was caused by variables that could not be measured in a lab. Their conclusion noted, "People are nourished by other people within an understanding community." This stance was long supported by developmental psychologists who held that humans are "wired for connectivity." This connectivity is what is exemplified by MI skills poignantly evidenced when married with the MI spirit.

SPIRIT AND PRACTICE

Given these conceptual underpinnings, how does the MI spirit evidence itself in a practical manner within our daily rehabilitation practice? As rehabilitation professionals, we strive to pursue a deeper understanding of our clients' values, motivations, and experiences without implicit and/or explicit judgment. This is realized in our practices where listening, understanding, support, and authenticity lie at the heart of our work. The adage "You have two eyes, two ears, and one mouth; use them in that ratio" is particularly apt here. It is our responsibility to appreciate the uniqueness of each of our clients, to understand the connotative meaning of their disabilities, and to offer the gift of time in spite of pressures otherwise. We strive to see the world through our clients' eyes, and through this process we have the possibility of collectively redefining, in spite of the particular disability, what is possible. Through listening, we strive to learn a new piece of information about our rehabilitative clients with each interaction and to take away more understanding as to who they are as unique individuals. The combination and balance of science/training/expertise of the clinician and a compassionate heart yields a clinical situation where authentic dialogue is possible. Without prejudgment, we enter our client contacts with open minds and open hearts. It is our belief that rehabilitation at its core is a relationship-based endeavor. Who among us does not wish to be heard, supported, validated, and understood? The MI spirit, coupled with MI skills, allows these client wishes to unfold—in a milieu where our clients can increasingly flourish.

READER REFLECTION QUESTIONS

Again, before moving on, let's take a moment to reflect:

- What are the signs that your spirit is intact?
- What contributes to your spirit being intact?
- What are the signs that your spirit has faded?
- What contributes to your spirit fading?
- How do you know when the team has lost the spirit?
- What helps you increase your spirit at work?
- What helps you increase your spirit at home?

Awareness and Roadblocks

As previously mentioned, Lequerica and Kortte (2010) present a model that describes the factors that promote effective rehabilitation. There is growing evidence that maximization of rehabilitation benefits requires the patient to be actively engaged in the process. While we readily recognize that acceptance, compassion, empowerment, and partnership can be effective tools to promote this engagement, the spirit can be misplaced or abandoned when confronted with roadblocks. These roadblocks can arise from the provider's burdens or stressors, from interactions with difficult patients or families, and from the environment or context of interactions. The frustrations with our own struggles or those of the patient or others in the environment can leaves us tired and reverting to less effective styles (e.g., directing) or losing our compassion or acceptance.

Gordon and Edwards (1997) have identified a series of verbalizations and behaviors that undermine effective communication and indicate our spirit is fading. These are described in Figure 1.2.

Perhaps a first step is realizing that we all have off days and lose our way. Demonstrating acceptance and compassion toward ourselves and our colleagues is a good beginning. Mindful self-awareness is useful in recognizing when we have lost our spirit. Reflecting and observing can help you answer these questions.

While our ability to fully realize and live in the MI spirit and values will never be perfect, there are steps we can take to support our efforts and the efforts of those around us. First, self-monitoring and self-awareness of signs we are losing our way and ongoing self-monitoring are key. Second, additional ongoing training in the form of workshops, readings, and peer supervision is useful in building strong habits that reflect key values and the MI spirit. While individual training is valuable, training of the entire team, service line, or organization can create an organization where values and skills are developed and ongoing maintenance of these attitudes and behaviors takes place. There is evidence that a wide range of healthcare providers including physicians, nurses, therapists, community health workers, nursing techs, and support personnel can learn and use these skills. Basic skills can be taught in cost-effective ways to reach the entire team and organization (www.HopkinsPEP. org). Third, creating and fostering a culture where these values are explicitly stated and reinforced by an entire organization provides a supportive context. Among other approaches, this can take the form of statements of values that are posted for the benefit of staff and patients, creation of patient/family advisory groups, or

1. Ordering, directing, commanding
2. Warning or threatening
3. Giving advice, suggestions, solutions
4. Persuading, arguing with logic, lecturing
5. Moralizing, preaching, using "should"
6. Disagreeing, judging, criticizing, blaming
7. Agreeing, approving, praising
8. Shaming, ridiculing, labeling
9. Interpreting, analyzing
10. Reassuring, sympathizing, consoling
11. Questioning, probing
12. Withdrawing, distracting, humoring changing subject

FIGURE 1.2 12 Roadblocks to Listening

development of peer mentoring programs that highlight the expertise of those with lived experience and partnership with them.

Summary

We will conclude by revisiting the team meeting interaction from the beginning of the chapter and then review the key takeaway points on spirit and values in MI. Examining the team dialogue, we can see where several team members have lost the spirit of MI as they encounter this challenging client situation.

> As a reminder, the team is meeting about a spinal cord injury patient who has been on the unit for some time. The team is dealing with, and talking about, a patient who has not grasped a main tenet of rehabilitation—that the patient needs to be an active participant in their care. The individual is reluctant to go to therapy, saying "If I rest, I will get better." They are reluctant to participate in self-care cathing and skin management and would like to eat in their room rather than participate in any group interaction. When asked to participate, they are often irritable and angry. The team members are discussing the situation and making comments: "This person isn't using our program. . . . It is frustrating that he doesn't do more . . . he has so much potential. . . . We need to set a strict behavioral plan and let him know what our rules are. . . . Maybe we need to just give him more time to get on board. . . . I think we need to educate him how if he doesn't do his self-cares he will have a lot of problems and can't go home and may need to go to a nursing home. . . . I think he is depressed and we need to do a diagnostic interview and perhaps start meds. . . . If he listened to us, then he would do better and would see progress."

How might the observations and comments be different if they were infused with MI spirit? We may see less judgment and more compassion—"What are the burdens this person is carrying?" We may see less focus on what we need to tell the patient and more "What does the patient know about the importance of skin checks?" We may see less emphasis on the patient listening to us and more us listening to them— "What are your long-term goals? How does bed rest get you there? What do you think your role should be in your recovery?" We may see less us–them and more collaboration/partnership—"We seem to all be on one side and the patient on the other. How do we build a collaboration?"

Patient–team struggles often arise when we are dealing with a challenging interaction and lose our spirit. An MI-consistent approach would be for the team to continue supporting one another and the patient by being mindful of when the spirit and values are lost and compassionately reminding ourselves or others to reconnect to the foundational values and spirit.

Key Takeaways

- The rehabilitation setting is an ideal environment for the practice of MI as the two share similar philosophies, spirit, and values.
- Communication styles may be classified into directing, following, or guiding based on the relative balance of asking, listening, and informing. The guiding style helps us avoid some traps and pitfalls that undermine the therapeutic alliance, prevent progress, and reduce patient/provider satisfaction. In the light of conversational styles, MI can be conceptualized as "refined guiding" in that it involves a purposeful conversation, using balanced conversational elements to elicit the patient's own arguments for change and engagement. It is style that is effective in rehabilitation and chronic care environments.
- Avoiding the fixing reflex and developing an approach infused with MI spirit and skills helps address ambivalence and avoid pushback ("yes, but . . ."). It has the added benefit of reducing clinician frustration and moving the patient more quickly to action. It is helpful to remember, MI is less like bulldozing and more like gardening.
- The spirit of MI is marked by: *acceptance*: Rogerian unconditional positive regard, withholding judgment, supporting autonomy and the right to choose, demonstrating accurate empathy; *compassion*: giving priority to another's needs, being mindful of the burdens they carry; *empowerment*: seeking understanding and valuing their goals and perspectives, recognizing their strengths; and *partnership*: not "to" but "with," combining the health expertise of the professional with the person's expertise of themselves and their situation, avoiding the "expert trap."
- In the MI world there are a number of acronyms that can help remind us of key elements. One of these is ACE = P (for acceptance + compassion + empowerment = partnership), to remind us of the spirit. Another is RULE:
  Resist the fixing reflex
  Understand your client's motives
  Listen
  Empower your client
- You can review the values and spirit of MI and see more examples at www.rehabilitationengagementcollaborative.org.

Final Questions for Discussion and Further Exploration

1. How do the philosophy and skills of MI fit with the practice of your discipline?
2. What skills do you already see in your patient interactions?
3. Based on the philosophy and skills of MI, what would you like to see more of in your interactions with patients and colleagues?
4. What would you do less of to make your style more MI-consistent?

References

Asay, T. P., & Lambert, M. J. (1999). The empirical case for the common factors in therapy: Quantitative findings. In M. A. Hubble, B. L. Duncan, & S. D. Miller (Eds.), *The heart and soul of change: What works in therapy* (pp. 23–55). American Psychological Association. https://psycnet.apa.org/record/1999-02137-001

Dali Lama 14th (2023, November 17). Words of Truth. https://www.dalailama.com/teachings/words-of-truth.

Engel, G. L. (1977). The need for a new medical model: A challenge for biomedicine. *Science, 196*(4286), 129–136.

Frankel, V. (2006). *Man's search for meaning.* Beacon Press.

Fromm, E. (1956). *The art of loving.* HarperCollins.

Gordon, T., & Edwards, W. S. (1997). *Making the patient your partner: Communication skills for doctors and other caregivers.* ABC-CLIO.

Institute of Medicine. (2001). *Crossing the quality chasm: A new health system for the 21st century.* National Academy Press.

Jackson, S. W. (1992). The listening healer in the history of psychological healing. *American Journal of Psychiatry, 149*(12), 1623–1632.

Kohut, H. (1971). *The analysis of the self.* University of Chicago Press.

Lequerica, A. H., & Kortte, K. (2010). Therapeutic engagement: A proposed model of engagement in medical rehabilitation. *American Journal of Physical Medicine & Rehabilitation, 89*(5), 415–422.

Miller, W., & Rollnick, S. (2002). *Motivational interviewing: Preparing people for change* (2nd ed.). Guilford Press.

Miller, W. R., & Rollnick, S. (2009). Ten things that motivational interviewing is not. *Behavioural and Cognitive Psychotherapy, 37*, 129–140.

Miller, W., & Rollnick, S. (2013). *Motivational interviewing: Helping people change* (3rd ed.). Guilford Press.

Miller, W. R., & Rollnick, S. (2023). *Motivational interviewing: Helping people change and grow.* Guilford Publications.

Nietzsche, F. (2019). *Human, all too human: A book for free spirits.* https://plato.stanford.edu/entries/nietzsche/. First Published in 1818.

Pascal, B. (1670). Pensées. https://www.gutenberg.org/cache/epub/18269/pg18269.txt

Prochaska, J. O., & DiClemente, C. C. (1992). Stages of change in the modification of problem behaviors. In M. Hersen, R. M. Eisler, & P. M. Miller (Eds.), *Progress in behavior modification* (Vol. 28, pp. 183–218). Sycamore Publishing Company.

Reik, T. (1975). *Listening with the third ear: The inner experience of a psychoanalyst.* Farrar, Straus and Giroux.

Rogers, C. R. (1967). The interpersonal relationship: The core of guidance. In C. R. Rogers & B. Stevens (Eds.), *Person to person: The problem of being human* (pp. 89–118). Real People Press.

Rogers, C. R. (1980). *Way of being.* Houghton Mifflin.

Rogers, C. R. (1995). *On becoming a person: A therapist's view of psychotherapy.* Mariner Books.

Rollnick, S., & Miller, W. R. (1995). What is motivational interviewing? *Behavioural and Cognitive Psychotherapy, 23*, 325–334.

Schechter, N., Butt, L., Jacocks, C., Staguhn, E., Castillo, R., & Wegener, S. T. (2021). Evaluation of an online motivational interviewing training program for rehabilitation professionals: A pilot study. *Clinical Rehabilitation, 35*(9), 1266–1276. https://doi.org/10.1177/02692155211002958

Schontz, F. C., & Fink, S. L. (1957). The significance of patient–staff rapport in the rehabilitation of individuals with chronic physical illness. *Journal of Consulting Psychology, 21*(4), 327–334.

Trieschmann, R. (1980). *Spinal cord injuries: Psychological, social and vocational adjustment.* Pergamon Press.

Wolf, S. (1966). Mortality from myocardial infarction in Roseto. *Journal of the American Medical Association, 195*(2), 186.

Wright, B. (1960). *Physical disability: A psychological approach.* Harper & Row Publishers.

2 Application of Motivational Interviewing in the Rehabilitation Environment

AN OVERVIEW

Katherine S. Wright and Charles H. Bombardier

Introduction

In many ways, motivational interviewing (MI) is synchronistic with the values and practices of rehabilitation, particularly through the common emphasis on patient-centered care. Patient-centered care has been defined by the Institute of Medicine as "'care that is respectful of and responsive to individual patient preferences, needs, and values'" and that ensures "that patient values guide all clinical decisions" (Barry & Edgman-Levitan, 2012, p. 780). MI is completely consistent with patient-centered care, and patient-centered care is at the heart of the rehabilitation process.

The spirit of MI, which drives the approach, is one of full focus on patient needs and preferences. As discussed in Chapter 1, the four key elements of the spirit are partnership, acceptance, compassion, and empowerment. Each one of these elements puts the patient at the center of the approach, such that in the partnership element between the healthcare provider and patient, the provider is collaborating as an expert with the patient, who is equally an expert on themselves. With the acceptance element of the MI spirit, the healthcare provider brings to this collaboration a

Katherine S. Wright and Charles H. Bombardier, *Application of Motivational Interviewing in the Rehabilitation Environment* In: *Motivational Interviewing in Medical Rehabilitation*. Edited by: Nicole Schechter, Connie Jacocks, Lester Butt, and Stephen T. Wegener, Oxford University Press. © Oxford University Press 2024. DOI: 10.1093/oso/9780197748268.003.0003 respect for a patient's autonomy and a genuine interest in understanding a patient's perspective. The element of compassion brings the pursuit of the patient's best interest to all interactions. Lastly, the element of empowerment orients the healthcare provider to a strengths-based approach, assuming that the patient already has the motivation and resources within themselves and that these strengths can be brought to awareness and lead to action (Miller & Rollnick, 2023). When patients enter a rehabilitation program, their success will depend on the team engaging them as partners and leaders in their care, and the spirit of MI can set the tone for true patient-centered care and partnership.

The spirit of MI parallels many of the foundational value-laden beliefs and principles articulated by Beatrice Wright (1983), whose writings are especially studied by rehabilitation psychologists. In particular, the notions that every individual needs respect and encouragement, that the rehabilitation team must attend to (*evoke*, in MI terms) the person's assets, that rehabilitation should be tailored to the unique characteristics (e.g., goals) of the individual, and that the team must understand the person's phenomenological perspective all dovetail nicely with MI spirit.

Alternatively, there are aspects of rehabilitation practice and values that may conflict with the spirit and methods of MI. Much about rehabilitation practice is directive and didactic in nature. It can pose a challenge to integrate MI practices into treatments that depend on teaching and training patients and families. In rehabilitation where patients have experienced declines in important functional abilities, it may be easy to think that they "should" be motivated and ascribe little importance to interpersonal or other contextual factors that might influence patient engagement. More than once, rehabilitation therapists have shared that they "don't get paid to do counseling." The conflict here may come down to job description, professional identity, or perhaps doubts about one's competence in other styles of communication. In some cases, there may be pressure from insurance or managed care companies and/or an institution's expectations to demonstrate rapid patient progress, especially during inpatient rehabilitation programs. This pressure can push therapists toward more directive treatment approaches based on the assumption that MI may just take too long. For this reason, when training rehabilitation therapists to use MI, it is essential to demonstrate MI's efficacy.

Another area where the spirit of MI can collide with deeply held rehabilitation values has to do with the goal of rehabilitation being functional independence. Rehabilitation care teams in the United States often strongly value independence, which is consistent with a more individualistic culture. Indeed, the way that rehabilitation goals are framed centers on the level of assistance someone may need in any given task with the goal of achieving independence. Functional Independence Measure scores have been used for care planning and quality measurement for decades (Heinemann et al., 1993). These concepts are deeply embedded in justification for and accreditation of rehabilitation programs.

However, patients may have different cultural perspectives, individual beliefs, and value levels of dependence or interdependence that may conflict with the culture of a rehabilitation program. By taking an MI approach, the team would prioritize a patient's values, and this orientation to the patient's perspective may result in patients choosing goals that involve less independence and perhaps more collectivism. Fortunately, high-functioning rehabilitation teams make concerted efforts to understand patient values and goals at the outset of treatment and work toward aligning their functional goals with the patient's priorities.

Potential Benefits to Using MI in Rehabilitation

Perhaps the most important reason for rehabilitation teams to consider utilizing MI has to do with improving patient participation in therapies and adherence to treatment. As in every other field of medicine, patient adherence to recommendations and treatment within rehabilitation is limited. Nonadherence rates are likely in the 25%–35% range for rehabilitation therapies (Forkan et al., 2006). How actively patients participate during therapy sessions they attend is also variable. The average patient early in inpatient rehabilitation does not finish all exercises and participates passively rather than actively (Lenze et al., 2004). How actively patients with stroke and spinal cord injury (SCI) participate in rehabilitation therapies predicts important functional outcomes, including discharge destination and return to work or school (Lenze et al., 2004; Ozelie et al., 2012; Teeter et al., 2012). Therefore, it is desirable for rehabilitation programs not only to foster therapy attendance but also to maximize participation in therapy sessions.

There is a growing body of research demonstrating that MI interventions can play a role in improving therapy attendance, progress, and participation. In perhaps the most rigorous study to date, Vong and colleagues (2011) randomly assigned physical therapists (PTs) to a general communication training program or to an MI training program, after which the investigators observed outcomes in the chronic low back pain patients treated by these two groups. The investigators observed that patients treated by MI-trained PTs performed their home exercise program twice as often as the group treated by PTs who received standard communication training. Patients treated by MI-trained PTs also reported greater improvements in proxy efficacy, working alliance, treatment expectancy, lifting capacity, and health-related quality of life relative to controls. A meta-analysis of 14 studies that examined the effects of adding MI training to PTs showed that patients treated by MI-trained therapists demonstrated significantly greater self-efficacy and lower activity limitations (McGrane et al., 2015).

In the rehabilitation psychology literature, there is evidence of the efficacy of MI in certain areas. MI-based interventions have been used to increase health-promotion behaviors and physical activity to treat depression in people with multiple sclerosis (Bombardier et al., 2013) and to reduce depression in people with traumatic brain injuries (TBIs; Bombardier et al., 2009). A meta-analysis found that MI, when used with other rehabilitation approaches, resulted in significant immediate medium to very large improvements in multiple physical, psychological, social, and behavioral outcomes (Dorstyn et al., 2020). Of course, the rehabilitation-specific literature is overshadowed by the extensive body of research on the efficacy of MI in other medical and psychological treatment contexts (Frost et al., 2018).

The benefits of MI can be felt by the whole team. Another important reason to use MI in rehabilitation settings is that MI training has been shown to improve staff satisfaction and perceived cohesion (Pollak et al., 2016) and may also reduce staff burnout by decreasing patient disengagement (Endrejat & Kauffeld, 2021). Healthcare providers may often feel the pull to "correct" or "fix" a patient's problem, which the creators of MI term the *fixing reflex* (Miller & Rollnick, 2023). This pull may be accompanied by anxiety and concern about the patient, especially when the patient is making decisions with which the provider does not agree. However, MI emphasizes a patient-centered perspective, and when a provider reorients to a patient's goals and motivation, the provider can let go of some of the responsibility to fix or change something and may feel that the anxiety that accompanies the fixing reflex is alleviated. A mismatch of goals between the provider and patient often increases a patient's resistance to change. But when goals are aligned and resistance, or talk that sustains current behavior, decreases the whole encounter may be more enjoyable for all involved.

Perceived Barriers to Using or Learning MI

There is evidence that rehabilitation team members do not already use MI. For instance, McGrane and colleagues (2015) found that PTs are not routinely trained in evidence-based strategies to motivate patients and do not provide systematic motivational interventions. Thus, strategies are needed to scale up MI training. However, this investment of time for training can be daunting, given the demands already placed on rehab teams, in addition to a number of other perceived barriers that providers have raised. Table 2.1 describes types of concerns that may come up when providers are considering an MI training and trying to determine if MI will be useful in their work.

TABLE 2.1

Perceived Barriers to Using or Learning MI

Barriers/Myths about MI	Reality
"Motivation to change resides within the patient, and there's nothing I can do about that."	Motivation does reside in the patient, but research on communication styles shows that healthcare providers can make a difference by eliciting and enhancing people's motivation to change (Patterson & Forgatch, 1985).
"My job is to educate and give advice, and then it is up to them—education is not enough to change behavior or get patients to their goals."	Education alone may not be enough to change behavior and achieve goals. However, when education is provided in an MI-consistent way, it can be included throughout the behavior change process to enhance goal-oriented behavior. For instance, education may support patients resolving ambivalence about change as they learn more about the pros and cons of a specific behavior. Once goals are identified, they are more likely to be achieved when people set implementation intentions (specify "the when, where, and how of responses leading to goal attainment"; Gollwitzer, 1999, p. 494) than when they only state goal intentions. Strategically using education to help patients when they are identifying their implementation intentions will help providers increase patients' success and change behavior (Gollwitzer, 1999).
"Sometimes patients say they want to do something, but then they don't follow through. Words are cheap!"	Research shows that follow through on goals improves when goals are specific, are more proximal, and have a positive outcome (vs. goals that are vague, distal, or based on the absence or prevention of a behavior; Gollwitzer, 1999). If we hear more vague language, we can help patients tailor goals to make them more attainable. Research has sought to analyze the strength and directness versus passivity of a person's verbal commitments to make changes. In a study examining patients' language during MI sessions focused on substance use, commitment strength was predictive of proportion of days abstinent, thus demonstrating that a patient's words do hold weight (Amrhein et al., 2003). A patient's language may also signal how important they consider this goal or how confident they are to achieve it. Listening for clues about importance or confidence will help a provider identify the potential barriers to change and focus the conversation.

(continued)

TABLE 2.1 *Continued*

Barriers/Myths about MI	Reality
"I already have developed my communication style that works for me."	Communication style is highly personal and feels like part of our identity/personality, so it can be threatening to examine the strengths and weaknesses of something so personal. MI training mostly sharpens and organizes skills people already know are good practice, such as listening, demonstrating empathy, and accurately reflecting the patient's experience.
"Open-ended questions take too long. It opens the door for an extremely verbose patient to start talking forever!"	Providers tend to perceive patients to be talking longer than they are. A study of physician behavior showed that they were interrupting patients within an average of 18 seconds of the first concern described (Beckman & Frankel, 1984). There is a place for both closed-ended questions and open-ended questions. Open-ended questions can be used strategically throughout an encounter to elicit information (particularly at the start of a visit, prior to providing any education, and at the end of a visit to elicit any last questions). In the instances when patients do become verbose, reflections and summaries can be used to guide the conversation.
"MI is a strategy that only psychologists can do."	Anyone can learn MI strategies, and research shows that many disciplines of healthcare providers and others are successful in using this approach to help their patients (Amrhein et al., 2003). Additionally, research has not identified any relationship between ability to learn MI and years of graduate education (Miller et al., 2004).
"Patient communication is about style, not science."	It is both about style and backed up by science. There are more than 40 years of research on MI demonstrating its effectiveness in increasing patient motivation and facilitating behavior change. For instance, a meta-analysis of MI's efficacy in healthcare settings found that MI showed a moderate advantage over other approaches for a variety of behavioral issues in healthcare, including HIV viral load, dental outcomes, death rate, body weight, alcohol and tobacco use, sedentary behavior, self-monitoring, confidence in change, and approach to treatment (Lundahl et al., 2013).

TABLE 2.1 *Continued*

Barriers/Myths about MI	Reality
"Patient counseling is not my job, not what I do, and I don't get paid for it."	This is counseling with a small *c*. Talking with patients, and motivating them, is part of nearly every healthcare provider's job. Making small tweaks and integrating some MI strategies into how we approach everyday conversations may help. Behavior change is a process that takes time, and patients may be guided through that process with multiple providers in different ways. MI can be used like a relay race; where you leave off with a patient, another provider can pick up with the patient in the next encounter.
"My patients are all compliant."	If this is true, change would be easy, and our patients would be reaping the gains! However, there is ample research documenting varying levels of noncompliance when people are asked to take up a new health behavior change. For example, Sluijs and colleagues (1993) studied a sample of physical therapy patients who were prescribed an exercise program. The 41% of this sample who reported not following through with the program identified the reasons for noncompliance as (1) barriers perceived and encountered, (2) lack of positive feedback, and (3) feelings of helplessness. MI strategies help providers help patients identify barriers to change and ways in which they can increase their confidence and problem-solve around the barriers, increasing their likelihood of succeeding.
"If I am only seeing a patient once or even just a couple times, what's the point?"	MI strategies have been shown to be effective and promote change in even single doses (Bein et al., 1993). In most cases, behavior change is achieved via a process that cannot be short-changed. Think of MI as facilitating a relay race, with each provider helping the patient move through the process of change across visits. One provider may help move the patient out of the phase of preintention, so now the patient is open to considering change; the next provider may help the patient work through weighing the pros and cons of change and work through ambivalence; and so on. Change takes time, and people often must "recycle" phases of change before ultimately following through. If a provider moves a patient even a bit forward in their confidence to make a change during a session, they have succeeded. Every visit is a valuable opportunity.

Note: MI = motivational interviewing.

READER REFLECTION QUESTIONS

Before moving forward, take a moment to reflect:

- What are the benefits to you of using MI in your work context?
- What are the barriers to you of using MI in your work context?
- How confident are you, on a scale of 1 to 10, that you might be able to use MI in your work context?
- What makes you so confident?
- How important is it to you, on a scale of 1 to 10, that you might be able to use MI in your work context?
- What makes it so important?
- What are some things that might help improve your confidence and/or importance?

Rehabilitation and Health Behavior Change

Rehabilitation is largely about health behavior change, and MI fits well with evidence-based theoretical models for health behavior change. These models can function as a behavior change roadmap, while MI strategies help the provider guide the patient forward.

One popular model, the health action process approach (HAPA), divides health behavior change into three phases: *preintenders*, *intenders*, and *actors* (Schwarzer et al., 2011). Preintenders are not ready to change the target behavior. To form intentions to change, they must understand and care about the risks of the status quo (risk perception), must believe that the target behavior can meaningfully reduce the risk (outcome expectancy), and have confidence that they can perform the target behavior (task self-efficacy). Intenders are ready to act. To do so, they need to form an action plan, determine how they will cope with barriers to change, and identify a way to sustain any new behaviors. In the last phase, actors have started to change their behaviors. Once action has begun, the person needs ongoing work to address barriers to maintaining their new behavior and to plan how they will cope with inevitable relapses.

MI strategies can be used to understand where a patient is within these theoretical constructs of readiness for change and relative to a particular health behavior, as well as to assist the person to move logically in the direction of change. For instance, a rehabilitation therapist might approach the topic of skin care with a patient with recent SCI by asking a strategic open-ended question to gauge their place on the roadmap, such as "What do you already know about taking care of your skin after

SCI?" If the patient is a preintender, the therapist can ask the patient follow-up open-ended questions about the theoretically relevant constructs, including risk perception, such as "What have your doctors and therapists told you about the need to pay special attention to your skin?" Outcome expectancy can be investigated with a question like "From what you know already, what are the most effective ways of preventing skin problems?" Task self-efficacy can be assessed with "How confident are you that you could perform pressure reliefs every 15 minutes when in your wheelchair if you decided to do that?" Alternatively, if the patient does not yet have relevant knowledge, and after getting the patient's permission, the clinician can use the MI technique *Ask-Offer-Ask* to offer information about risks, efficacy, and ease of carrying out key prevention strategies.

By using MI principles and strategies and using HAPA as a roadmap, the therapist can ensure that their conversations with patients match their patients' readiness for change and avoid common mistakes. The most common mistake is for the therapist to assume the patient is an intender or actor when they are still a preintender and not yet ready for change. As an example, the therapist might focus on action-planning (e.g., "We need to discuss how to do pressure reliefs every 15 minutes when you are in your wheelchair") when the patient does not yet understand their risk of developing pressure ulcers and before they have formed an intention to do pressure reliefs. When the provider pushes for an action plan before the patient is ready, this can lead to interpersonal tension and resistance as well as avoidable failure experiences.

Overestimating readiness can also have repercussions for the patient's future healthcare visits. The provider might have documented that the patient was committing to a certain plan, such as daily skin checks; and when the patient arrives at the next appointment and no progress has been made on this plan, the next provider may interpret this as nonadherence or noncompliance. Now the patient has been labeled in the next note as having failed, when they were not yet ready to make the change in the first place. By accurately identifying and then documenting a patient's readiness for change, the provider is not only helping the patient succeed but also helping other providers understand where to pick up next in the behavior change process. For instance, if the provider documents that the patient is an intender and still weighing the hassles of daily skin checks against the benefits of detecting red spots before they turn into pressure ulcers, the next provider will know what to expect and where to start the conversation.

Another way these behavior change conversations can go awry is when the clinician is overly reliant on teaching or advising. Teaching and giving unsolicited advice are known to generate patient resistance, especially when the patient is not ready for action (e.g., "Now I want to tell you why you need to do pressure reliefs every 15 minutes"). Using an MI approach, the clinician can instead use open-ended questions, reflections, and summaries to elicit and reinforce desire, ability, reasons, and need statements as a prelude to eliciting commitment language (i.e., intention to change). Specifically, one can elicit concerns about the status quo (e.g., "From what you have learned so far, why does the rehab team worry so much about people doing pressure reliefs?"). Similarly, an eliciting approach can be used to identify ways in which the targeted health behavior would mitigate risk (e.g., "How do skin checks help to prevent getting pressure sores?"). This approach may also instill confidence that the patient is capable of engaging in skin checks by asking a question like "If you decided to do skin checks, how would you fit them into your daily routine?" MI strategies simply represent an eliciting approach to achieving the HAPA behavior change process goals.

AMBIVALENCE ABOUT CHANGE

With regard to phase of change, MI will be particularly helpful with intenders—the patients who are still contemplating change and feeling ambivalent about this choice. While the provider's reasons for the proposed change are clear to them, it may not be clear to the patient, who has a competing reason for not engaging in the change that may be equally compelling. In these cases, it may be easy to make assumptions about the patient's values or beliefs (e.g., "They don't seem to care about their health!"). However, in most cases, patients very much care about their health, but they may not fully understand the importance of the change, it may not seem like the right time to change, or they have tried to change in the past and now have little confidence in their ability to change. MI can enable a real exploration of the barriers and give the provider a much more nuanced understanding of a patient's situation and how to help.

It is easy when a patient's goals and motivation align with the provider's goals. However, this is not always the case as patients have their own priorities and past experiences that color their readiness for change. As opposed to a phase model of change, an even simpler way to conceptualize readiness for change may be viewing that change on a continuum of *not ready*, *unsure*, or *ready*. Indeed, the majority of patients likely fall into the *unsure* or *ambivalent* section of the continuum. When patients are ambivalent, using an MI approach can help them explore uncertainty and give voice to their reasons or beliefs for attempting or avoiding change. Patients are pleasantly surprised when providers are interested in understanding things from their point of view through questions like "So while we know doing pressure reliefs is critical to your health, we also know there are barriers to doing them. What would be your main barriers to doing pressure reliefs while up in your wheelchair?"

In rehabilitation, there are many potential targets for change about which patients may feel ambivalent, and so there are many opportunities for rehabilitation team members to use MI. In an inpatient rehabilitation setting, perhaps a patient is ambivalent about requesting and waiting for assistance to get out of bed. Or perhaps a patient may be uncertain about their ability to transfer from one surface to the next. Maybe a patient is uncertain about trying a new medication. In the outpatient rehabilitation environment, a patient may feel ambivalent about returning to work. They may feel uncertain about their readiness for neuropsychological testing. Or perhaps they are not sure about joining the amputee peer support group. Across the continuum of rehabilitation settings, there is no lack of opportunities for patients to make changes, and thus MI can be useful across all of these different settings.

READER REFLECTION QUESTIONS

Before moving forward, take a moment to reflect:

- What kinds of health behaviors are your patients trying to change?
- Do you often encounter preintenders, intenders, or actors?
- How do you communicate differently with preintenders, intenders, or actors?

Strategic Times to Use MI in Rehabilitation With a Patient

Whether change is the focus of the interaction or not, bringing the MI spirit (partnership, acceptance, compassion, and empowerment) to interactions with patients will likely enhance these visits for both the healthcare provider and the patient. However, there are specific situations when MI may be particularly helpful.

AT THE START OF A VISIT

Taking an MI approach to the start of a visit can set a positive and empowering tone. MI begins with the assumption of partnership with a patient and fostering their autonomy. This approach can be incredibly powerful for patients in rehabilitation settings as they have often undergone a traumatic or significant change in their level of functioning or health status and, as a result, may be experiencing a loss of control. An MI approach seeks to empower the patient through a strengths-based focus and communicates respect for their agency. Particularly with neurological injuries, patients are often experiencing their bodies differently, relearning how their body functions, and building trust in their bodies again.

One MI technique that is especially useful at the start of the visit is asking permission. Given that patients may feel powerless and lack control in a healthcare setting, beginning the interaction by asking permission to discuss a particular topic quickly increases the patient's sense of control over the conversation and lowers resistance.

Additionally, beginning a visit with an open-ended question can empower the patient and be efficient for the provider. Using an open-ended question like "What is your priority for today's visit?" will ensure that the patient's questions are addressed. This also allows the provider to plan the episode of care and avoids a power struggle over topic priorities.

BEFORE PROVIDING EDUCATION

Patients often enter rehabilitation settings with a new diagnosis, and part of the rehabilitation process is to learn about their new condition, self-management, and how this condition will impact other areas of their lives and health. Education will likely be a significant part of each interaction with their rehabilitation team members, and these educational opportunities can be both streamlined and maximized with the use of MI. As rehabilitation progresses, MI strategies can be uniquely useful to reinforce what a patient has learned in their therapy sessions and to build on that knowledge base across disciplines.

An MI approach to education encourages providers to focus on the patient's experience and knowledge base, guided by the spirit of partnership and empowerment. To achieve this, providers can elicit from patients what they already know, which does six critical things: (1) it will help providers gain an understanding of a patient's knowledge base, (2) it will identify any gaps or misconceptions in this knowledge, (3) it will reinforce patients' memory and understanding of the information, (4) it may save the provider time when information does not have to be repeated, (5) it avoids irritating a patient and damaging rapport if a provider is not repeating something they already know, and (6) it may increase a patient's confidence in what they have learned. One provider's education may also overlap with what another discipline is teaching, so this strategy can serve to reinforce or generalize learning across different contexts.

BEFORE PROVIDING TEST RESULTS OR FEEDBACK

Providing feedback regarding test results or diagnoses offers another opportunity for education and an occasion to first elicit what a patient may already know about the condition or to learn what they were expecting to hear about the outcome of the test or procedure. Having this information from the patient first allows providers to tailor their update to the patient's level of understanding and expectations. This may change the level of detail they provide or prepare for an emotional reaction that may take additional time to process.

An MI approach will also help guide the flow of the remainder of the interaction and help a provider determine how the new information is getting consolidated. After providing the update or new diagnosis, the MI strategies of using open-ended questions and reflections will help a provider better understand how the patient is interpreting the results and integrating this information into what they already knew. For instance, saying something like "I know that was a lot of information I just provided. Tell me what you heard," will elicit much more information than a closed-ended question, such as "That was a lot of information; do you understand?" Without providing an opportunity for the patient to paraphrase or ask questions, assumptions are easily made about someone's level of understanding and potentially create or compound misunderstandings and risks, damaging the patient–provider relationship. Alternatively, by coming alongside the patient and learning their perspective, a provider can enhance the relationship by communicating genuine interest and concern.

WHEN A BARRIER TO ENGAGEMENT IN REHABILITATION IS IDENTIFIED

When rehabilitation team members see a patient who is not fully engaged, MI offers a framework for exploring the potential barrier in a nonjudgmental way. On the inpatient rehabilitation unit, signs of reduced engagement may look like wanting to stay in bed when therapy is scheduled or declining medications or other nursing care activities. In the outpatient rehabilitation clinic setting, signs of low engagement may show up as a patient being chronically late for therapy appointments or not participating in any of the home exercise plan or other homework. In any setting, it may be that cognitive deficits, mood disorder, or a substance use disorder is interfering with engagement and participation in rehabilitation tasks. The MI spirit sets up a provider to take a collaborative stance and to elicit and explore a possible barrier with genuine curiosity and compassion. Then, when the barrier is identified, MI strategies can be used to assess the patient's readiness to address this barrier and weigh the pros and cons of behavior change.

AT THE END OF A SESSION BEFORE SETTING GOALS OR ASSIGNING HOMEWORK

As a session is ending, providers usually have a goal or homework assignment in mind. However, as MI is patient-centered, this approach can guide providers toward a goal or assignment that is both meaningful to the patient and achievable. Providers could use an open-ended question to elicit from the patient what they would like to work on outside of session. This could also look like suggesting homework and then using MI strategies to assess the patient's perceived importance of doing this task as well as their confidence that they can accomplish this outside of session.

Application of MI to Conditions Commonly Found in Rehabilitation

Given the types of clinical conditions that complicate rehabilitation, such as cognitive impairment, mood disorders, and substance use disorders, MI techniques seem especially well suited as an adjunct to standard rehabilitation. MI-consistent therapist behaviors seem to engage multiple neurobiological structures and functions that are vital to cognitive rehabilitation (Feldstein Ewing et al., 2011). MI can be used to engage people in mental health treatment, which seems especially important in a setting where people may not be overtly seeking or wanting such treatment (Holt et al., 2017). MI was developed for substance use disorders, and rehabilitation represents an excellent window of opportunity to begin addressing these conditions as well (Bombardier et al., 1997).

MOOD DISORDERS

Mood disorders are also common in rehabilitation settings, especially depression. Depression is highly prevalent and disabling in people with TBI, stroke, Parkinson's disease, and multiple sclerosis (Conroy et al., 2020). MI can be used by medical providers to increase the likelihood that affected persons will seek mental health services (Holt et al., 2017). For providers in rehabilitation settings who treat mental health disorders (most likely psychologists or social workers), MI can enhance outcomes when combined with another active treatment, such as cognitive behavioral therapy (Marker & Norton, 2018; Romano & Peters, 2015). Please review Chapter 8 for more information on this topic.

SUBSTANCE USE DISORDERS

Addiction is another common comorbid condition found in patients in rehabilitation settings. The rate of substance use can be higher in rehabilitation patient populations than in the general public. For instance, a recent meta-analysis reported that 35% of people with TBI had premorbid alcohol abuse and 34% had preinjury other drug abuse (Unsworth & Mathias, 2017). MI-based interventions have been well established and validated in the treatment of addiction, with the strongest evidence in the treatment of tobacco and alcohol abuse or dependence, particularly when designed as a brief intervention (DiClemente et al., 2017). Please review Chapter 9 for more information on this topic.

COGNITIVE IMPAIRMENT

Cognitive impairment is one of the most common types of impairment in rehabilitation settings. Cognitive deficits can be obvious and expected among patients with TBI or stroke or subtler and more unexpected as in people with SCI or limb loss related to peripheral vascular disease. Therefore, an important question to address is whether MI is feasible and effective to use in people with cognitive impairment. Please review Chapter 10 for more information on this topic.

Applications of MI Outside of Direct Patient Encounters

Less research has been published in the area of using MI in organizations, professional relationships, or families. Nevertheless, it is relatively easy to imagine how core MI concepts and strategies might be applied in these other contexts. The MI spirit, including partnership, acceptance, compassion, and empowerment, is an aspirational feature of how interprofessional peers seek to work together and represents a good principle for relating to trainees and subordinates as well. In this section, we explore some of these nonclinical applications of MI within rehabilitation practice more broadly.

MI IN CONSULTATIONS WITH INTERDISCIPLINARY PEERS

Using the MI spirit and methods can work well when consulting with multidisciplinary team members because MI begins with a deep respect for the knowledge, experience, and perspectives of others. This leads to a focus on asking open-ended questions and a more thorough understanding of what the consultee needs, what has already been tried, and what the consultee is willing to do. This more deferent style is particularly important with nurses, who are on the front lines of patient care and typically have a host of important observations. Asking questions about what has already been tried or what seems to have had partial success before jumping to giving advice communicates respect to the consultee and grows the relationship through empathic listening. This sort of exploration provides opportunities to reflect or affirm consultee strengths in regard to how they have managed the problem thus far, ultimately fostering a greater sense of self-efficacy in the consultee. Optimally, the MI eliciting style can lead to the consultee identifying how they may change their strategy or find alternative solutions to explore. Like with patients, when the consultee is the one to identify new options, they are more likely to implement the alternatives. Please see Chapter 6 for more information about this topic.

MI AS A FRAMEWORK FOR LEADERSHIP WITHIN A TEAM OR SYSTEM

When the rehabilitation team needs to make changes, team leaders could approach the team in huddles or rounds with these same principles in mind. A team leader who demonstrates openness to each team member's experience by eliciting feedback, listening, and then accurately reflecting the various opinions or considerations raised, with careful attention to emotional valence in the room, can help the team come to agree on alternative solutions.

Groups and organizations show many of the same patterns of behavior change as individuals, in that a system may or may not be ready for a specific change. Without identifying the pros and cons to change, communicating effectively across the group, addressing barriers to change, and moving forward with a solution that is acceptable to stakeholders/team members, change is unlikely to be successful. Leadership may find that change occurs more smoothly across the rehab team when the team's level of readiness matches the task. For instance, just as moving too fast with an individual patient and rushing a solution or change plan may set the patient up for failure, the team may benefit from additional discussion if a significant proportion of the team is still ambivalent about the need for change or their confidence in their ability to make the change. Please see Chapter 6 for more information about this topic.

MI WITH FAMILY SYSTEMS

For many patients, having positive social support and helpful family systems can improve their engagement in the rehabilitation process across the continuum of care (McCauley et al., 2001; Tomberg et al., 2007). However, families can be similar to rehab teams in that change is likely not going to be successful if all members are not on board. For instance, in family conferences in the inpatient rehabilitation setting, a discharge plan may seem completely clear to the rehab team, given the patient's progress and resources. However, it will be important to assess the level of readiness of the family system to accept such a discharge plan. If they have a different understanding of their resources, or if they feel less confident that they could provide the level of assistance and caregiving the team is asking of them, the rehab team is going to encounter resistance. That resistance should signal to the rehab team that more time needs to be spent resolving that ambivalence. Please review Chapter 11 for more information on this topic.

MI IN SUPERVISORY RELATIONSHIPS

Across disciplines in rehabilitation, models of training and education often include clinical teaching and tiered models of supervision. When looking at supervisory relationships, many of the same principles of using MI with consultees can be applied to interactions between supervisors and trainees. Likewise, a supervisor may find the same scenarios they encounter with patients also occurring with trainees, such as a trainee feeling resistant to making a change.

When examining the training guidelines for many rehabilitation disciplines, it may be the case that these guidelines inherently include the spirit of MI. For instance, in the health service psychology field, the guidelines for clinical supervision include the following assumptions: "occurs within a respectful and collaborative supervisory relationship" and "uses a developmental and strength-based approach" (American Psychological Association, 2015, p. 35). To make the trainee–supervisor relationship more collaborative and strength-based, these guidelines advocate for the use of an MI-consistent information-sharing strategy called Ask-Offer-Ask.

To use Ask-Offer-Ask, the supervisor would inhibit their impulse to immediately share their opinions and instead, take additional time to elicit the trainee's own clinical observations and reasoning (e.g., "If you were to give yourself advice about this case, what would you say are your options and the best way forward?"). The act of recalling, generalizing, and reasoning from prior experience reinforces the skills needed for independent practice and builds confidence. If the trainee satisfactorily articulates the options and best plan, the supervisor only needs to reinforce the trainee's sound treatment-planning skills. If something is left out or if there is an aspect of the plan with which the supervisor disagrees, they ask the trainee for permission to provide some additional ideas. After providing additional or corrective input, the supervisor finishes by eliciting from the trainee what they take away from the supervisor's input as it pertains to management of the case, as well as gauging the trainee's readiness to set a goal for incorporating this feedback or implementing a change. The use of this strategy assumes that the trainee already has an adequate fund of knowledge and experience and that the supervisor discusses the reasons for adopting a different supervisory process with the trainee beforehand. When this strategy is not employed and a supervisor offers solutions immediately, they run the risk of the trainee becoming a relatively unengaged, passive recipient of information and advice.

READER REFLECTION QUESTIONS

Before moving forward, take a moment to reflect:

- In what contexts would you like to use MI in your work? With patients? Families? Team members? Supervisees?
- What is one way you might incorporate MI into that context?

Summary

In summary, MI both is consistent with rehabilitation values and can help promote the behavior change and goals of rehabilitation. So much is asked of patients during a rehabilitation program, and there is often a lot of change required as part of learning the management of a new condition. Broadly, research on adherence to a variety of recommendations across a range of treatment settings worldwide shows that approximately half of all medical patients do not fully adhere to physicians' advice (World Health Organization, 2003). Using MI strategies has been shown to help patients resolve ambivalence about health behavior change as part of the management of their new neurological/physiological condition and to increase the likelihood of behavior change in a patient-centered way that will facilitate their engagement in rehabilitation across the continuum of settings.

Luckily, MI can be learned by any type of provider in a rehabilitation setting, and the more providers who are bringing the MI spirit to interactions, the smoother and more satisfying these interactions will be for patients, families, and the rehabilitation team alike. Training programs in MI have been shown to be effective in increasing providers' use of these strategies, and with regular boosters, multidisciplinary teams can deliver the basic skills of MI and are more likely to facilitate behavior change.

Application of the MI spirit and strategies does not have to be limited to patient interactions; bringing this approach to situations in which change is being proposed for supervisees, family units, or perhaps whole rehab teams can help individuals feel heard, barriers be identified, and the group feel more cohesive and aligned during a decision-making and change process. MI is not about convincing anyone to change; rather, "MI is about arranging conversations so that people talk themselves into change, based on their own values and interests" (Miller & Rollnick, 2013, p. 4). The partnership between patients and their rehabilitation providers has always been critical to helping patients meet their rehabilitation goals, and MI can enhance this partnership for better outcomes.

References

American Psychological Association. (2015). Guidelines for clinical supervision in health service psychology. *American Psychologist, 70*(1), 33–46.

Amrhein, P. C., Miller, W. R., Yahne, C. E., Palmer, M., & Fulcher, L. (2003). Client commitment language during motivational interviewing predicts drug use outcomes. *Journal of Consulting Clinical Psychology, 71*(5), 862–878.

Barry, M. J., & Edgman-Levitan, S. A. (2012). Shared decision making—The pinnacle of patient-centered care. *New England Journal of Medicine, 366*(9), 780–781.

Beckman, H. B., & Frankel, R. M. (1984). The effect of physician behavior on the collection of data. *Annals of Internal Medicine, 101*, 692–696.

Bein, T., Miller, W., & Tonigan, J. (1993). Brief interventions for alcohol problems: A review. *Addiction, 88*, 315–335.

Bombardier, C. H., Bell, K. R., Temkin, N. R., Fann, J. R., Hoffman, J., & Dikmen, S. (2009). The efficacy of a scheduled telephone intervention for ameliorating depressive symptoms during the first year after traumatic brain injury. *Journal of Head Trauma Rehabilitation, 24*(4), 230–238.

Bombardier, C. H., Ehde, D. M., Gibbons, L. E., Wadhwani, R., Sullivan, M. D., Rosenberg, D. E., & Kraft, G. H. (2013). Telephone-based physical activity counseling for major depression in people with multiple sclerosis. *Journal of Consulting and Clinical Psychology, 81*(1), 89–99.

Bombardier, C. H., Ehde, D., & Kilmer, J. (1997). Readiness to change alcohol drinking habits after traumatic brain injury. *Archives of Physical Medicine and Rehabilitation, 78*(6), 592–596.

Conroy, S. K., Brownlowe, K. B., & McAllister, T. W. (2020). Depression comorbid with stroke, traumatic brain injury, Parkinson's disease, and multiple sclerosis: Diagnosis and treatment. *Focus, 18*(2), 150–161.

DiClemente, C. C., Corno, C. M., Graydon, M. M., & Wiprovnick, A. E. (2017). Motivational interviewing, enhancement, and brief interventions over the last decade: A review of reviews of efficacy and effectiveness. *Psychology of Addictive Behaviors, 31*(8), 862–887.

Dorstyn, D. S., Mathias, J. L., Bombardier, C. H., & Osborn, A. J. (2020). Motivational interviewing to promote health outcomes and behaviour change in multiple sclerosis: A systematic review. *Clinical Rehabilitation, 34*(3), 299–309.

Endrejat, P. C., & Kauffeld, S. (2021). Learning motivational interviewing to preserve practitioners' well-being. *International Journal of Workplace Health Management, 14*(1), 1–11.

Feldstein Ewing, S. W., Filbey, F. M., Hendershot, C. S., McEachern, A. D., & Hutchison, K. E. (2011). Proposed model of the neurobiological mechanisms underlying psychosocial alcohol interventions: The example of motivational interviewing. *Journal of Studies on Alcohol and Drugs, 72*(6), 903–916.

Forkan, R., Pumper, B., Smyth, N., Wirkkala, H., Ciol, M. A., & Shumway-Cook, A. (2006). Exercise adherence following physical therapy intervention in older adults with impaired balance. *Physical Therapy, 86*(3), 401–410.

Frost, H., Campbell, P., Maxwell, M., O'Carroll, R. E., Dombrowski, S. U., Williams, B., Cheyne, H., Coles, E., & Pollack, A. (2018). Effectiveness of motivational interviewing on adult behaviour change in health and social care settings: A systematic review of reviews. *PLOS ONE, 13*(10), Article e0204890.

Gollwitzer, P. M. (1999). Implementation intentions: Strong effects of simple plans. *American Psychologist, 54*(7), 493–503.

Heinemann, A. W., Linacre, J. M., Wright, B. D., Hamilton, B. B., & Granger, C. (1993). Relationships between impairment and physical disability as measured by the Functional Independence Measure. *Archives of Physical and Medical Rehabilitation, 74*, 566–573.

Holt, C., Milgrom, J., & Gemmill, A. W. (2017). Improving help-seeking for postnatal depression and anxiety: A cluster randomised controlled trial of motivational interviewing. *Archives of Womens Mental Health, 20*(6), 791–801.

Lenze, E. J., Munin, M. C., Quear, T., Dew, M. A., Rogers, J. C., Begley, A. E., & Reynolds, C. F. (2004). The Pittsburgh Rehabilitation Participation Scale: Reliability and validity of a clinician-rated measure of participation in acute rehabilitation. *Archives of Physical Medicine and Rehabilitation, 85*(3), 380–384.

Lundahl, B., Moleni, T., Burke, B. L., Butters, R., Tollefson, D., Butler, C., & Rollnick, S. (2013). Motivational interviewing in medical care settings: A systematic review and meta-analysis of randomized controlled trials. *Patient Education and Counseling, 93*(2), 157–168.

Marker, I., & Norton, P. J. (2018). The efficacy of incorporating motivational interviewing to cognitive behavior therapy for anxiety disorders: A review and meta-analysis. *Clinical Psychology Review, 62*, 1–10.

McCauley, S. R., Boake, C., Levin, H. S., Contant, C. F., & Song, J. X. (2001). Postconcussional disorder following mild to moderate traumatic brain injury: Anxiety, depression, and social support as risk factors and comorbidities. *Journal of Clinical and Experimental Neuropsychology, 23*(6), 792–808.

McGrane, N., Galvin, R., Cusack, T., & Stokes, E. (2015). Addition of motivational interventions to exercise and traditional physiotherapy: A review and meta-analysis. *Physiotherapy, 101*(1), 1–12.

Miller, W. R., & Rollnick, S. (2013). *Motivational interviewing: Helping people change* (3rd ed.). Guilford Press.

Miller, W. R., & Rollnick, S. (2023). *Motivational interviewing: Helping people change and grow* (4th ed.). Guilford Publications.

Miller, W. R., Yahne, C. E., Moyers, T. B., Martinez, J., & Pirritano, M. (2004). A randomized trial of methods to help clinicians learn motivational interviewing. *Journal of Consulting Clinical Psychology, 72*(6), 1050–1062.

Ozelie, R., Gassaway, J., Buchman, E., Thimmaiah, D., Heisler, L., Cantoni, K., Foy, T., Hsieh, C.-H. J., Smout, R. J., Kreider, S. E. D., & Whiteneck, G. (2012). Relationship of occupational therapy inpatient rehabilitation interventions and patient characteristics to outcomes following spinal cord injury: The SCIRehab project. *Journal of Spinal Cord Medicine, 35*(6), 527–546.

Patterson, G. R., & Forgatch, M. S. (1985). Therapist behavior as a determinant for client noncompliance: A paradox for the behavior modifier. *Journal of Consulting Clinical Psychology, 53*(6), 846–851.

Pollak, K. I., Nagy, P., Bigger, J., Bilheimer, A., Lyna, P., Gao, X., Lancaster, M., Watkins, R. C., Johnson, F., Batish, S., Skelton, J. A., & Armstrong, S. (2016). Effect of teaching motivational interviewing via communication coaching on clinician and patient satisfaction in primary care and pediatric obesity-focused offices. *Patient Education and Counseling, 99*(2), 300–303.

Romano, M., & Peters, L. (2015). Evaluating the mechanisms of change in motivational interviewing in the treatment of mental health problems: A review and meta-analysis. *Clinical Psychology Review, 38*, 1–12.

Schwarzer, R., Lippke, S., & Luszczynska, A. (2011). Mechanisms of health behavior change in persons with chronic illness or disability: The health action process approach (HAPA). *Rehabilitation Psychology, 56*(3), 161–170.

Sluijs, E. M., Kok, G. J., & van der Zee, J. (1993). Correlates of exercise compliance in physical therapy. *Physical Therapy, 73*(11), 771–782; discussion 783–786.

Teeter, L., Gassaway, J., Taylor, S., LaBarbera, J., McDowell, S., Backus, D., Zanca, J. M., Natale, A., Cabrera, J., Smout, R. J., Kreider, S. E. D., & Whiteneck, G. (2012). Relationship of physical therapy inpatient rehabilitation interventions and patient characteristics to outcomes following spinal cord injury: The SCIRehab project. *Journal of Spinal Cord Medicine, 35*(6), 503–526.

Tomberg, T., Toomela, A., Ennok, M., & Tikk, A. (2007). Changes in coping strategies, social support, optimism and health-related quality of life following traumatic brain injury: A longitudinal study. *Brain Injury, 21*(5), 479–488.

Unsworth, D. J., & Mathias, J. L. (2017). Traumatic brain injury and alcohol/substance abuse: A Bayesian meta-analysis comparing the outcomes of people with and without a history of abuse. *Journal of Clinical and Experimental Neuropsychology, 39*(6), 547–562.

Vong, S. K., Cheing, G. L., Chan, F., So, E. M., & Chan, C. C. (2011). Motivational enhancement therapy in addition to physical therapy improves motivational factors and treatment outcomes in people with low back pain: A randomized controlled trial. *Archives of Physical Medicine and Rehabilitation, 92*(2), 176–183.

World Health Organization. (2003). *Adherence to long-term therapies: Evidence for action.* Retrieved July 8, 2021, from https://apps.who.int/iris/bitstream/handle/10665/42682/924 1545992.pdf

Wright, B. A. (1983). *Physical disability: A psychosocial approach* (2nd ed.). Harper and Row.

3 Motivational Interviewing Communication Skills

Nicole Schechter and Stephen T. Wegener

Introduction

This chapter presents the motivational interviewing (MI) tasks, tools, and skills that can be used to make the spirit come alive (see Chapter 1), and in particular those that are helpful in the rehabilitation context. In this chapter we will introduce foundational MI skills, overview the role language plays in behavior change, and outline how particular skills can be applied to specific tasks and phases of MI.

For a more in-depth, comprehensive review of MI tasks and skills, please refer to Miller and Rollnick's *Motivational Interviewing: Helping People Change and Grow* (2023). You can also learn more at https://www.rehabengage.org/, a resource constructed by the book's editors to provide guidance on putting MI skills into practice in the rehabilitation context. It is important to state at the start of this chapter that the spirit of MI is its foundation, so unless that is in place, even the most accurately used MI tool/skill will have limited effectiveness.

Let's look at the situation discussed in Chapter 1 with some slight adjustments. This time, instead of focusing on the team's interactions, we will focus on the interaction between one rehabilitation team member and the patient:

Nicole Schechter and Stephen T. Wegener, *Motivational Interviewing Communication Skills* In: *Motivational Interviewing in Medical Rehabilitation*. Edited by: Nicole Schechter, Connie Jacocks, Lester Butt, and Stephen T. Wegener, Oxford University Press.

A person with spinal cord injury has been on the unit for some time. The individual is reluctant to go to physical therapy and occupational therapy, saying "If I rest, I will get better." He is reluctant to participate in self-care, catheterization, and skin checks and would like to eat in his room rather than participate in any group interaction. When asked to participate, he is often irritable and angry. The therapy team has given significant education about the importance of self-care, and the patient just does not seem to care. The physician has explained all the negative health outcomes that can occur if he develops a pressure sore, but this has not made any difference. The psychologist has talked with the patient about depression and the importance of behavioral activation as a treatment for depression, with no effect. The patient continues to state that he wants to rest.

As you read through this chapter, reflect on how the skills discussed are or are not reflected in what the team has tried thus far. We will revisit this example and see how the patient's ambivalence might be addressed more effectively with attention to MI tasks and skills.

Foundational MI Skills

MI emphasizes four core communication skills that when used effectively, in conjunction with the MI spirit, help to engage the patient, establish partnership, and guide patients toward change. These skills—open-ended questions, affirmations, reflections, and summaries—are referred to by their acronym: OARS. Appropriately, OARS help a practitioner in the same way that boating oars help a boater (Figure 3.1). OARS help the practitioner move the patient forward, backward, speed up, slow down, or change course.

OPEN-ENDED QUESTIONS

Open-ended questions can be defined simply as questions that cannot be answered with a "yes" or "no." In MI, open-ended questions serve a few important purposes: (1) encourage patient elaboration and mobilize change talk, (2) give the patient a sense

O = Open-Ended Questions
A = Affirmations
R = Reflections
S = Summaries

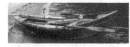

FIGURE 3.1 Foundational MI Skills

of control over the conversation, (3) convey practitioner interest in the patient's experience and thoughts, (4) create an activated patient, and (5) avoid the passive question–answer trap.

Open-ended questions cannot be answered with a *yes* or a *no*. They may begin with words like *What, How*, and *Tell me about*. Though the word *why* begins questions that cannot be answered with *yes* or *no*, MI encourages practitioners to avoid this question-starter because it is more likely to elicit a defensive patient response secondary to its potential parental tone. When asked "Why" questions, patients may perceive that the practitioner is questioning their experience and therefore may feel the need to defend their positions. This moves a patient away from change and toward maintaining the status quo.

Open-ended questions can be used at any point in the patient–practitioner interaction. It is recommended that during the early phases of establishing the professional relationship, open-ended questions are general; and as the MI tasks progress, they become more targeted to help the patient focus and move in a particular direction.

Many practitioners worry that when general open-ended questions are used the patient will become circumstantial or tangential and that time will be wasted. In fact, a study by Singh Opsina and colleagues (2019) showed that, on average, general medicine practitioners interrupted patients after 11 seconds of talking. Interestingly, the literature suggests that most patients without a significant cognitive impairment, if uninterrupted, will talk for no more than 30 seconds in a general medicine setting and no more than 90 seconds in a specialty medicine setting (Beckman & Frankel, 1984; Blau, 1989; Langewitz et al., 2002; Marvel et al., 1999).

Even so, it is not recommended to use only open-ended questions during an interaction with a patient. In fact, MI recommends balancing open-ended questions with reflections in a ratio of 1:2. That is, for every one open-ended question that is asked, provide two reflections. This pattern also helps avoid the question–answer communication trap that is very common when using closed-ended questions. Please see Chapter 10 for how it may be important to adapt open-ended questions when working with special populations such as a person with a traumatic brain injury.

A practitioner might consider using open-ended questions at the beginning of an encounter and at the end of an encounter. At the beginning of an encounter, one might ask "What would you like to accomplish during our time together?" and at the end of an encounter, "What questions do you have about what we have discussed?" or "What do you see as the best next step?" Open-ended questions are also very useful when mobilizing change talk: "What makes you consider this particular goal?" See Table 3.1 for examples of open-ended questions in rehabilitation contexts.

TABLE 3.1

Foundational MI Skills

Foundational MI skill	Patient statement	Example provider response
Open-ended question	I did it (bowel program)—I didn't like it, but I did it.	Tell me one thing that went well.
	I'm in so much pain. I'm here, but I don't know how much I'm going to be able to do.	What have you already tried today to help your pain?
	Everyone keeps telling me PT is important. I just want to rest, but I'll do it once because my son wants me to. That's it though.	What do you think your son is hoping will happen if you do PT?
Affirmation	I did it (bowel program)—I didn't like it, but I did it.	You were scared to try the bowel program today, and you did it anyway. You are brave.
	I'm in so much pain. I'm here, but I don't know how much I'm going to be able to do.	You made it to our appointment today despite pain. You are committed to getting stronger.
	Everyone keeps telling me PT is important. I just want to rest, but I'll do it once because my son wants me to. That's it though.	You've decided to do PT because your son wants you to do it. You care deeply about your family.
Reflection	I did it (bowel program)—I didn't like it, but I did it.	You were scared to try the bowel program today, and you did it anyway.
	I'm in so much pain. I'm here, but I don't know how much I'm going to be able to do.	You made it to our appointment today despite pain.
	Everyone keeps telling me PT is important. I just want to rest, but I'll do it once because my son wants me to. That's it though.	You've decided to do PT today.
Summary	I did it (bowel program)—I didn't like it, but I did it.	You were feeling anxious about the bowel program. You found a way to do it anyway. What do you think the next step should be?

(*continued*)

TABLE 3.1 *Continued*

Foundational MI skill	Patient statement	Example provider response
	I'm in so much pain. I'm here, but I don't know how much I'm going to be able to do.	On the one hand, you're in a ton of pain. On the other hand, you are here in the office. What is one thing you'd like to accomplish today?
	Everyone keeps telling me PT is important. I just want to rest, but I'll do it once because my son wants me to. That's it though.	You'd like to rest. and at the same time your son and others want you to do PT to get stronger. Where does that leave you?

Note: MI = motivational interviewing; PT = physical therapy.

AFFIRMATIONS

Affirmations can be defined as recognitions and acknowledgments of "that which is good," including the individual's inherent worth as a fellow human being (Miller & Rollnick, 2013). It is important to differentiate affirmations from compliments or statements of praise like "Great job today" or "I am proud of you." Such statements, though positive, infer that the deliverer is an authority figure and in a position to judge the recipient. Affirmations are strongest when they do not reference the practitioner (using the word *I*) but rather focus entirely on the patient (using the word *You*). When used in this way, affirmations help to build rapport, build confidence, reduce defensiveness, and promote self-efficacy in the long term. According to Linehan et al. (2002), affirmations can also support patient retention in treatment.

Since affirmations are comments about an individual's behavior, intention, internal strength, or power, they are only effective when delivered genuinely. This does not necessarily mean that you need to know a patient very well to provide an affirmation. In fact, affirmations are appropriate for use during any phase of the professional relationship. Practitioners using affirmations in the earlier stages of the professional relationship will need to choose them thoughtfully after careful listening and observation and use them sparingly to avoid over-reaching. If the affirmation does not feel sincere to the practitioner, it should not be said.

Affirmations come in many forms. They may identify a patient's behavior or intention, like "You didn't get to do the exercises four times this week, and you still did three—that was twice more than last week." Affirmations can also comment on a patient's strength or character, like "You have been through so much—you are resilient." Finally, affirmations may be less specific and instead describe an over-all appreciation for the person, like "You are committed." An affirmation can be thought of as having two parts—an observation of what the person has said or done and an inference about an enduring strength or quality of their character. Many find that an affirmation "formula" can be useful: patient's behavior/words + character-istic or personal quality. See Table 3.1 for examples of affirmations in rehabilitation contexts.

REFLECTIONS

Reflection is the primary listening skill in MI and is sometimes referred to as *active listening*. This skill, especially when accompanied by nonverbal cues and body lan-guage, like eye contact and facial expressions that match the patient's emotional state, can quickly facilitate connection with a person. *Reflections* can be defined as statements that describe what the speaker means. Three benefits of reflections are that they (1) demonstrate to the patient that you are listening intently, (2) encour-age the patient to continue talking and exploring, and (3) decrease sustain talk and discord or limit the risk of increasing the patient's defensiveness. Using reflections of emotion, in MI known as *accurate empathy*, is a very useful skill when patients are frustrated or upset.

Reflections may be *simple*, a restatement of the patient's thought or reuse of a key word that the patient used, or *complex*, a statement that infers what the patient means. Practitioners unfamiliar with MI often worry that simple reflections will sound like they are parroting the patient and that their complex reflections will be wrong and put off patients. Interestingly, reflections are very unlikely to make conversations feel unnatural. Since complex reflections are guesses, there is a risk that the guess could be wrong. However, most patients respond to an inaccurate complex reflection by overtly correcting the practitioner (e.g., "That's not it—I'm not worried, I'm terrified"), which further connects the patient and practitioner. For practitioners who would prefer to be conservative with complex reflections, it can be helpful to "undershoot" a guess about the patient's emotional state. That is, instead of reflecting that the patient is *devastated*, the practitioner may opt for the word *disappointed*.

While reflections are recommended to be the most frequently used skill in each of the four MI tasks, studies of practitioners untrained in MI show that reflections are far outnumbered by questions 1:10 (Miller & Rollnick, 2013). Ideally, two or three reflections should follow each question asked. As practitioners become more comfortable using reflections, this ratio will be easier to achieve.

SUMMARIES

A *summary* is considered a distinct MI skill; however, it can be conceptualized as a set of reflections that consolidate what the patient has described over the course of the conversation. Summaries can be used in any MI task and at any point in the patient–practitioner encounter. The main purposes of a summary are to (1) convey that the practitioner has been listening, (2) encourage the patient to reflect on their own experiences and provide opportunity for additional input from the patient, and (3) highlight specific topics to strengthen patient motivation.

There are three different types of summaries: collecting, linking, and transitional. A *collecting* summary tends to follow an open-ended question that prompts a patient to list out experiences, thoughts, or attributes. For example, a practitioner might ask a patient about what they have tried to manage low back pain in the past, guiding the patient to identify several past experiences. A collecting summary reflects the patient's treatment experiences and asks for additional ideas.

A *linking* summary connects a comment the patient makes to something that they have said in the past as a way to reflect an important theme, like "You described today being really scared that the exercises will exacerbate your pain. I remember last week you mentioned you were afraid to go on a walk with your wife because you were worried about making pain worse."

A *transitional* summary is the type that most people think of when they hear the word *summary* in that it helps to wrap up the encounter or move to a different topic within the same encounter. This type of summary helps to consolidate the patient's memory for what was discussed during the session and/or ensures that patients feel validated before moving the conversation on due to time limitations. Of course, the practitioner can decide at the end of the encounter whether the patient or the practitioner should do the summary. With a patient with reasonable cognitive capacity, it can be helpful for the practitioner to ask the patient, "From your perspective, what are the key takeaways from today's session? What do you see as the next steps?" This approach reflects a respect for the patient as partner and can provide the practitioner with information as to what the patient understands and plans to do. The practitioner may need to add to the patient summary in a respectful manner consistent with the collaborative spirit of MI.

One of the most strategic uses of summaries involves summarizing the patient's uncertainty about change or engagement in care. When done effectively, these summaries reflect a "zoomed out" picture of both sides—the reasons to avoid and the reasons to engage, in this order. These summaries allow a patient to take a step toward appreciation of their situation. They also demonstrate the practitioner's MI spirit in that they convey a nonjudgmental and respectful view of the patient.

MI Communication Skills: Getting to Change Talk

SUSTAIN TALK

In working with patients, families, or even team members, there can be reluctance to change or ambivalence about engagement in rehabilitation and healthcare behaviors. This is a natural part of the change task. First, let's address how reluctance or ambivalence is often reflected in inconsistent behaviors or in the language people use. In these situations, we expect to hear what in MI is referred to as *sustain talk*. This sustain talk is marked by reasons to maintain the status quo or not adopt new behaviors. People may talk about reasons that they don't think they need to, or can't, change. Some examples are "I would like to exercise more but . . . ," "I don't need to learn to use the wheelchair, soon I will get my strength back," and "That might work for others but not for me." Higher levels of sustain talk are related to lower levels of individual change, so reducing sustain talk is critical in moving toward change (Magill & Hallgren, 2019). How do we respond when we hear people using sustain talk? Several guiding principles are useful, and their implementation relies on our foundational MI OARS skills. Our response should be guided by (1) acknowledgment of what the person is saying and not asking questions that would lead to more sustain talk (a reflection such as "You are uncertain whether you need to learn how to use the wheelchair" reflects the patient's ambivalence and does not ask the person to justify their behavior or statement with more sustain talk) and (2) exploration of the situation by using open-ended questions that encourage exploration of change rather than maintaining status quo—"What would it be like or mean for you if you did try the wheelchair?" It is likely there will be ongoing sustain talk; however, we are looking to reduce the amount of sustain talk and increase the change talk. Let's now explore change talk and how it can be fostered.

WHAT IS CHANGE TALK?

Change talk occurs when a patient uses language that indicates they are considering or ready to live differently or modify their health behavior. How do we recognize change talk? MI uses an acronym, DARN-CAT, to remind us of the different types of change talk people use. People may describe the *desire* to change, *ability* to change, *reasons* to change, or *need* for change. DARN is preparatory language that, when used, suggests someone is considering and preparing for a change. CAT stands for *commitment*, *activation*, and *taking steps* toward change. CAT is implementation language that, when used, suggests someone is beginning to act on change. When individuals use any change talk, the likelihood of them acting on a change increases

(Amrhein et al., 2003). Therefore, a primary responsibility for practitioners is to listen for, reinforce, and strategically mobilize change talk.

When you hear DARN-CAT, it is important to reinforce it to grow motivation by using OARS. Open-ended questions can be used to invite the patient to elaborate on the change talk. Remember that the more change talk the patient hears themselves use, the more likely they are to act. Therefore, asking questions like "In what ways might you . . ." or "How are you going to do that?" or "Tell me some examples of . . ." will strategically guide the patient to speak more about change. Affirmations can be used to validate, encourage, and grow confidence for making change. When a patient feels more confident in their ability to make change, they will be more likely to do so. Therefore, using affirmations like "You are someone who commits and follows through" or "You deeply care about your family and do your best to make them proud" will be helpful (Table 3.2).

Reflections can be used as another method for the patient to hear their own change talk and are likely, like questions, to prompt a patient to say more. The patient speaks in favor of change, they hear you repeat their language, and then they hear themselves speak in favor of change again. Summaries can be helpful especially when a patient is describing many aspects of DARN-CAT. By selecting the most

TABLE 3.2

DARN-CAT

Change talk category	Common statement starters	Patient statement example
Desire	I want I wish I'd like	I wish I could be as organized as I used to be. I used to never miss appointments, and now it happens so often.
Ability	I can I could I am able to	There is no way I can go to the store on my own right now, but I guess I could ask my cousin to come with me.
Reason	This is why	My wife is so stressed with all of this. She is why I have to learn to be more independent.
Need	I need to I have to I must	I need to help my wife. She is stressed.
Commitment	I am going to	I am going to do my bowel program myself tonight.
Activation	I've started to I'm planning to	I've started to gather the equipment I need for the bowel program.
Taking steps	I did	I did the bowel program independently last night.

important, relevant, or newest aspects of change talk and emphasizing them using a summary, a practitioner can be selective in growing motivation for specific behaviors or specific aspects of health.

See below for a brief patient–practitioner interaction. See if, as you are reading, you can identify which aspects of DARN you are observing and then notice how OARS are used to reinforce and elaborate on change talk.

PATIENT: "You know, I am really sick of being here. I just need to get out of here and get back home." (Need)

PRACTITIONER: "You can't wait for a change of scenery." (Reflection)

PATIENT: "Not just a change of scenery, though. My family is stressed coming back and forth to see me here. At least if I'm home, it will take their stress away." (Reason)

PRACTITIONER: "You care deeply about your family." (Affirmation)

PATIENT: "Exactly—They mean everything to me. Then once I'm home, I can start to actually help again. I don't exactly know how that will work or what I'll do, but I know I want to help my wife out." (Desire)

PRACTITIONER: "You want to do anything you can to ease the burden on your wife." (Reflection) "What do you think she might need help with?" (Open-ended question)

PATIENT: "Well, I used to be the dinner prep person. She's the cook, but I do the prep—the recipe-finder, the chopping, the defrosting. That kind of thing. I could probably still do some of that now." (Abilities)

PRACTITIONER: "There are still ways for you to contribute." (Reflection). "What do you think we might do while you're here so you are able to contribute to dinner prep?" (Open-ended question)

PATIENT: "I know you told me there's a kitchen on the floor. Could we work on maneuvering around that during one of my sessions? I know it's not exactly like my kitchen at home, but it's a start."

MOBILIZING CHANGE TALK

When patients are experiencing ambivalence about making a change and you are hearing sustain talk and not hearing spontaneous offerings of change talk, it is helpful to use OARS and other strategic, more advanced MI skills to mobilize change talk. Remember that patients are unlikely to act until they are talking about change. In this next section, we will introduce a few advanced MI skills that can be used to mobilize change talk and thus increase readiness. This will not be comprehensive, and the reader is encouraged to refer to Miller and Rollnick's 2023 work and other training resources (https://motivationalinterviewing.org/) for more in-depth material.

LOOKING FORWARD AND LOOKING BACKWARD QUESTIONS

Looking forward and *looking backward questions* are tools that help a patient remember a time when they were engaging in healthy behaviors or self-management of medical conditions and help a patient envision a future if they were to make a change or what might happen if they were to stick with the status quo. Some key questions that prompt a patient to look backward are as follows:

- What were things like before your stroke?
- How did you manage your weight before your spinal cord injury?
- Tell me about a time when your health was going well for you. What were you doing during that time?
- What is different about the person you were 5 years ago and the person you are today? The good and the not so good?

Not all of these questions are going to be helpful for each patient; however, you can see how each question provides an opening for the patient to talk about things that were going well and things that were going less well in the past. When individuals talk about the past, it can highlight discrepancies between how they used to behave and how they are behaving now, which are likely to prompt desires, abilities, reasons, or needs to do things differently now.

Some key questions that prompt a patient to look forward are as follows:

- What will be the likely outcome if you keep relying on your husband for all of your bathing needs?
- How would your family react if you started to use your manual wheelchair?
- How will things be 3 months from now if you were to be successful with self-managing your bowel program?

Again, not all of these questions are going to be helpful for every patient, while at the same time, any one of these questions can help open the floor for patients to use change talk.

REMEMBERING SUCCESSES

When patients are "stuck" in ambivalence or being reluctant to change, it can be helpful to use a remembering-successes technique. This technique draws the patient's attention away from the present ambivalence. Not only do we ask the patient to look backward at successes, as we discussed above, but we use elaborating questions to have the patient dive deeply into a past success and describe the who, what, where, when, and whys of their success. When patients describe with great detail past successes, we can guide them to apply aspects of those experiences to their current situation. See below for some questions that can help a patient remember and elaborate on their successes:

- What is one thing that you have been successful at changing in the past, even if it's small?
- What prompted you to make this change?
- What did you do to get started making this change?
- What did you do to stick with your decision to make this change?
- What problems or obstacles did you run into? How did you get past them?
- How easy was it?
- How did you feel after taking that one step?
- How do you feel about it now?
- What other successes have you had?

READINESS RULERS

Scaling readiness for change is a useful technique to prompt the patient to talk about DARN and even begin to identify a plan (CAT), if appropriate. You can also use a ruler to gauge importance and confidence, which are the two factors that contribute to readiness. Figure 3.2 shows a visual depiction of the *readiness ruler*. When using this tool with a patient, you can show an image of a ruler to guide the conversation, or you can speak about the ruler without the visual.

See below for how a professional might use the readiness ruler to elicit DARN from a patient who is ambivalent about going on the community outing using her manual wheelchair.

> PRACTITIONER: "On a scale of 1 to 10, how ready are you to go on tomorrow's outing, 10 being completely ready and 1 being not at all ready?"
> PATIENT: "I'd say I'm about a 7."
> PRACTITIONER: "A 7, okay. What makes you a 7 ready instead of a 5 ready?"

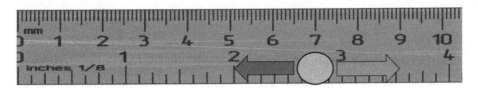

FIGURE 3.2 Readiness Ruler

PATIENT: "Well, I'm a 7 because I would love to get out of this place and see the world again. I need to remember that life isn't only about rehab and hospitals." (Need)

PRACTITIONER: "You are excited to get back to some of the places and activities you enjoyed before. (Reflection) What else makes you a 7 instead of a 5?"

PATIENT: "I've been working on navigating ramps in PT [physical therapy] and it's not going half bad. (Ability) Would be nice to see if it would actually work in the real world. (Desire) But, if it doesn't work . . . that would be pretty embarrassing."

PRACTITIONER: "You've been working hard. (Affirmation) You think it's time to test out your hard work."

PATIENT: "I guess it could be time (Ability), but it still makes me nervous."

PRACTITIONER: "What might help you move from a 7 to an 8 or 9 ready for this community outing?"

PATIENT: "Well I only have one more PT session between now and go time. I think if I could get two more sessions in so I could practice a little more . . . that would help."

PRACTITIONER: "You want to have more practice to build up your confidence a bit more. (Reflection) What do you think the next step should be?"

There are some key features of the conversation about the readiness ruler to notice here. First, all questions from the practitioner are open-ended. Second, once the patient's level of readiness is identified (7), the next question, "What makes you a 7 and not a 5?," guides the patient to talk about strengths and the DARN factors that motivate going on the community outing. This is a different approach than is typically used in healthcare, where there is a tendency to solely focus on the problem and how to move the person up the scale through problem-solving. Then, the professional uses the question "What might help you move from a 7 to an 8?" to guide the patient toward their own problem-solving task. Again, this is a different approach than is typically used, where we provide our own recommendations or ideas for how the patient might become readier for a change or a specific action. The readiness ruler strategy centers the patient as the driver of the ideas and the driver of the action plan. When the patient is the one to speak about change and then commit to change aloud, rather than us explaining all the reasons they should consider change and commit to change, we strengthen their motivation and likelihood to act.

READER REFLECTION QUESTIONS

Take a moment to reflect on how you usually respond to challenging cases, what skills and strategies you currently use, and how incorporating MI skills may help you be a more effective change agent.

- What do you do when you are met with a patient who is ambivalent or even resistant to making a change?
- How often do you spend time listening to change talk or mobilizing change talk from your patients before asking them or expecting them to make a change?
- Which of the mobilizing change talk techniques do you think could be useful in your work?
- Think about how one of your patients might react to these techniques?

MI Tasks

Now that we have explored foundational MI skills and how developing DARN-CATs is a key component in change, let's take get a big-picture view of the MI key task. MI consists of four essential relationship-building tasks that, when joined together, support a patient in making desired health changes. The four tasks build one on the other—*engaging, focusing, evoking,* and *planning.* Each task has distinct goals, different ways of using the motivational interviewing foundational skills, and varying therapeutic considerations that suggest when the relationship is ready for the next task.

The four tasks (see Figure 3.3) are organized in a specific order, which always begins with engaging. Sometimes the tasks move linearly; however, if at any point the work halts or plateaus, it is likely that returning to a previous task is indicated. In fact, it is common that practitioners need to return to the first task, engaging, at multiple time points over the course of treatment.

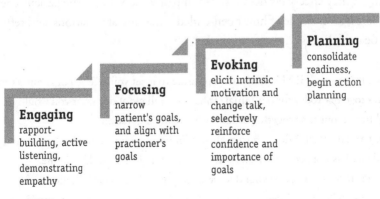

Engaging
rapport-building, active listening, demonstrating empathy

Focusing
narrow patient's goals, and align with practioner's goals

Evoking
elicit intrinsic motivation and change talk, selectively reinforce confidence and importance of goals

Planning
consolidate readiness, begin action planning

FIGURE 3.3 MI Tasks

ENGAGING

Engaging is the first task and is considered the "relational foundation." Engaging requires significant time and attention, perhaps more than the other task, as it builds the groundwork that allows MI to work effectively. When engaging, a practitioner completely appreciates the patient's values, goals, and perceptions. Though the practitioner might have their own treatment goals in mind, it is important in this phase that the practitioner prioritize hearing from the patient and avoid presenting their own agenda. A practitioner in this phase would steer away from prescribing the "right" way forward or a "recommended" treatment plan unless the patient clearly inquires.

The goals of the engaging task include the following:

- The patient feels comfortable and safe in the treatment environment.
- The patient feels comfortable and safe with the practitioner.
- The practitioner effectively demonstrates and communicates empathy toward the patient.
- The practitioner understands the patient's concerns, personal values, and goals for treatment and achieving self-defined quality of life.

Practitioners in this task will use all the basic MI skills in a nondirective manner. Open-ended questions can also be used to elicit the patient's concerns and hopes for treatment and demonstrate the practitioner's interest in learning about the patient above all else. Affirmations may be used to emphasize patient strengths, which will help to build patient self-efficacy for treatment. These can also help the patient to feel safe with the practitioner because they are accurately seeing the patient for who they are, including the barriers they have or are facing and the assets they intrinsically or extrinsically possess. Reflections are a very important strategy to use during engaging as they effectively demonstrate empathy and validate the patient's perspectives. Here is an example of how open-ended questions, affirmations, and reflections might be used during the engaging task.

PRACTITIONER: "Hi Mrs. Jones. It's a pleasure to meet you. We've got about 45 minutes together today for our initial evaluation. Tell me about what you would like to address in our time together today." (Open-ended question)

MRS. JONES: "Well, I don't exactly know. I'm having a lot of low back pain, and my balance has not been good lately. My doctor thought PT could help me."

PRACTITIONER: "You and your doctor are hoping PT can help." (Reflection)

MRS. JONES: "Right—I usually do what I'm told . . . by this doctor anyway. I want to feel better."

PRACTITIONER: "When you trust someone, you follow through on recommendations. You are committed to your health." (Affirmation)

MRS. JONES: "You got it. Not just my health . . . I have to get back into the swing of things!"

PRACTITIONER: "What will you be doing when you are back in the swing of things?" (Open-ended question)

FOCUSING

Focusing is the second task in MI, during which the practitioner guides the patient toward a desired change or a self-identified goal. At the beginning of treatment, a specific goal may be unclear either because the patient has many desired outcomes or because the patient is ambivalent about engaging in treatment in the first place. It is important that practitioners do not advance to the focusing task too early, falling into the "premature focus trap."

Once in the focusing task, patients may proceed very quickly, while for others this task will take considerable time. The goals of the focusing task include the following:

- Exploring multiple possible target behaviors or goals.
- Identifying one (or a few) target behaviors or goals on which to act.
- Outlining and agreeing upon concrete definitions of target behaviors and goals.
- Clarifying possible barriers and facilitators of the behavior/goal(s).

Practitioners in this task will use all the basic MI communication skills, perhaps with a greater emphasis on open-ended questions and reflections when identifying a session agenda or treatment goals. Open-ended questions can be used during this task to gauge the patient's readiness, sense of importance, and sense of confidence for different goals, as well as developing an understanding of the discrepancy between the patient's current behavior and desired behavior. Reflections will be helpful, as always, to demonstrate understanding of the patient's priorities. Summaries will also be particularly helpful once a target goal has been identified. Let's look at an example:

PRACTITIONER: "Hi Mrs. Jones. It's good to see you again. Today I was hoping to talk about some options for how we move forward with treatment. Would that be okay with you?"

MRS. JONES: "That sounds fine."

PRACTITIONER: "Alright. Last time you described having trouble with pain in your low back and balance. You identified how important it is to you to be able to take your granddaughter for walks in her stroller and mow the lawn. What did I miss?" (Summary, Open-ended question)

MRS. JONES: "Those are the two most important things. We also talked about me losing some weight and working on my nighttime sleep problems."

PRACTITIONER: "That's right. Four important goals: (1) going for walks with your granddaughter, (2) mowing the lawn, (3) losing weight, (4) improving sleep. What goal is most important to you right now?" (Open-ended question)

MRS. JONES: "Walking my granddaughter I think, though I'm just not sure how it's going to happen."

PRACTITIONER: "You're not certain how this will go. (Reflection) Help me understand more about these walks. How long do you want or need to be able to walk with your granddaughter and how many times per week?" (Open-ended question)

EVOKING

Evoking is MI's third task. A practitioner in the evoking phase will continue to use a guiding communication style to build the patient's motivation for the goal(s) that was identified during the focusing task.

The practitioner wants to avoid becoming too directive in telling the patient why they should be motivated for change, even though this may seem obvious given the practitioner's professional training and expertise. The optimal way to build internal motivation is for the patient to identify these themselves. The goals of the evoking task include the following:

- Elicit and strengthen change talk.
- Increase intrinsic motivation.

Practitioners in this task use all the foundational MI communication skills and more complex skills like asking permission and readiness rulers. Open-ended questions are useful during this task to get the patient talking about desires, abilities, reasons, and needs for change, as well as their sense of importance and confidence for the identified treatment targets. Reflections are used to convey understanding differently than in previous tasks, to strategically reinforce specific patient statements to strengthen motivation and quicken change. Though asking permission may be used during any task, it is particularly helpful when evoking if the practitioner wants to offer their own ideas around motivators. Asking permission helps us to avoid the "fixing reflex." The readiness ruler is an important skill during this task as it engages patients in a strategic conversation that typically strengthens motivation for change. Here is an evoking task example:

PRACTITIONER: "So walking with your granddaughter for about 20 minutes, twice per day, three days per week is what you'd like to target in our work together. Did I get that right?" (Summary)

MRS. JONES: "Yep. Still not sure how this is going to go, but yeah, I want to be able to do that."

PRACTITIONER: "You're nervous and it's still important to you. (Reflection) Tell me more about what makes this important to you?"

MRS. JONES: "Well this is my first grandchild, you know, and I have always told my daughter that I was going to be one of those active, involved grandmas. My mother wasn't like that at all for my kids, so I've always wanted to do it differently. That and my daughter works full-time so it would help her."

PRACTITIONER: "You wished your mother had been more involved with your kids (Reflection) and you are committed to being present for your grandkids now. You also care deeply about your daughter's well-being." (Affirmation)

MRS. JONES: "Of course! Nothing's more important than my family."

PRACTITIONER: "Would it be okay for me to add something to the reasons you've already described?" (Asking permission)

MRS. JONES: "Sure."

PRACTITIONER: "You've also mentioned a desire to lose weight. So though this goal isn't specifically about weight loss, it strikes me that walking more could help with that too. What are your thoughts?"

MRS. JONES: "That's very true. Another good reason."

PRACTITIONER: "At the same time that this is so important to you, you are worried. On a scale of 1 to 10, how confident are you that you can do these walks?"

PLANNING

Planning is the last MI task. Helpful indicators that it is time to move to the planning task include (1) when the patient has identified a clear goal, (2) finds it sufficiently important and are sufficiently confident that they can work on the change, and (3) have sufficient reasons for engaging in the behavior. If there is sustain talk, discord, or hesitation that arises regarding creating a change plan or if barriers are identified once a change plan is established, it may be necessary to revisit earlier tasks before proceeding with planning. The goals of the planning phase include the following:

- Action plan.
- Troubleshoot barriers to the action plan.
- Build skills.

Practitioners in this task continue using the guiding communication style with open-ended questions, affirmations, reflections, and summaries. Reflections are used to emphasize the patient's motivation and commitment. Open-ended questions then are used to elicit the patient's thoughts about an appropriate plan of action, solutions for barriers that arise once the action plan is in place, and what kinds of skills the patient needs to develop to carry out the plan. Affirmations highlight patient strengths that facilitate the action plan, and summaries are used to pull together and reiterate the plan or any determined plan changes. Asking permission and readiness rulers can be used in this task as they were in the evoking task. Here is an example:

PRACTITIONER: "So Mrs. Jones, you've identified that walking with your granddaughter is important to you because you want to be involved in her life, lose some weight, and help your busy daughter. (Reflection/Summary) What do you think the next step might be from here?" (Open-ended question)

MRS. JONES: "Well I'd love to be able to say that I can just get started with walking, but I'm too nervous about the balance."

PRACTITIONER: "Your sense is that we have to work on balance before you can safely start walking. (Reflection) You are very thoughtful about taking this step by step; you want to be successful." (Affirmation)

MRS. JONES: "Well yeah—Who wants to fail at their goals?"

PRACTITIONER: "What, if anything, has helped you with balance before?" (Open-ended question)

MRS. JONES: "I used to use a 3-point cane. That seemed to help, but I hated how I looked. I know that the doctor said you could teach me some balance exercises."

PRACTITIONER: "You're open to a cane, and you'd like to try some balance exercises. (Reflection) I can teach you two balance exercises today in our session, and then you can practice those at home between now and the next session. What do you think about that idea?" (Summary)

MRS. JONES: "That sounds good to me."

PRACTITIONER: "How many times per day and per week do you think you can start to practice these two exercises?" (Open-ended question)

MRS. JONES: "Maybe two times per day and 5 days a week."

PRACTITIONER: "So twice per day and 5 days a week. (Reflection) You believe doing the balance exercises will help you get to the point you can walk with your granddaughter which is your goal." (Reflection)

Summary

We have introduced the foundational MI skills, explored the role of language in behavior change, and outlined the tasks of MI. Let's return to the case example from the beginning of the chapter:

> A person with spinal cord injury has been on the unit for some time. The individual is reluctant to go to physical therapy and occupational therapy, saying "If I rest, I will get better." He is reluctant to participate in self-care, cathing, and skin checks and would like to eat in his room rather than participate in any group interaction. When asked to participate, he is often irritable and angry. The therapy team has given significant education about the importance of self-care, and the patient just does not seem to care. The physician has explained all the negative health outcomes that can occur if he develops a pressure sore, but this has not made any difference either. The psychologist has talked with the patient about depression and the importance of behavioral activation as a treatment for depression, with no effect. The patient continues to state that he wants to rest.

READER REFLECTION QUESTIONS

Ask yourself some questions:

- What MI skills would be helpful in these conversations?
- What language is the patient using? Change talk? Sustain talk?
- What task should the team be focusing on initially?

Key Takeaways

This case reminds us that there are many opportunities to use our MI spirit and skills:

- Use open-ended questions to understand the individual's perspective, affirm their honesty and desire to become more functional, reflect their emotion, summarize where they are and the options.
- Respond to the sustain talk by acknowledging the ambivalence. Look backward to explore how they overcame adversity and were successful in

the past, and look forward to explore what it might be like if they were to engage in the behavior. These approaches help identify strengths, DARN-CAT, and potential barriers.

- Rather than initially focusing on teaching and action planning, use OARS to engage and focus in on goals. Once that is established, explore options for achieving the goals. Prematurely attempting to talk the patient out of their initial idea or threatening them with negative consequences is likely to prolong the struggle rather than moving toward change.

When challenging patients and situations present, MI spirit and skills provide a way forward.

References

Amrhein, P. C., Miller, W. R., Yahne, C. E., Palmer, M., & Fulcher, L. (2003). Client commitment language during motivational interviewing predicts drug use outcomes. *Journal of Consulting and Clinical Psychology, 71*(5), 862–878.

Beckman, H. B., & Frankel, R. M. (1984). The effect of physician behavior on the collection of data. *Annals of Internal Medicine, 101*(5), 692–696.

Blau, J. N. (1989). Time to let the patient speak. *BMJ, 298*(6665), 39.

Langewitz, W., Denz, M., Keller, A., Kiss, A., Rütimann, S., & Wössmer, B. (2002). Spontaneous talking time at start of consultation in outpatient clinic: Cohort study. *BMJ, 325*(7366), 682–683.

Linehan, M. M., Dimeff, L. A., Reynolds, S. K., Comtois, K. A., Welch, S. S., Heagerty, P., & Kivlahan, D. R. (2002). Dialectical behavior therapy versus comprehensive validation therapy plus 12-step for the treatment of opioid dependent women meeting criteria for borderline personality disorder. *Drug and Alcohol Dependence, 67*(1), 13–26.

Magill, M., & Hallgren, K. A. (2019). Mechanisms of behavior change in motivational interviewing: Do we understand how MI works? *Current Opinion in Psychology, 30*, 1–5.

Marvel, M. K., Epstein, R. M., Flowers, K., & Beckman, H. B. (1999). Soliciting the patient's agenda: Have we improved? *JAMA, 281*(3), 283–287.

Miller, W. R., & Rollnick, S. (2013). *Motivational interviewing: Helping people change.* Guilford Press.

Miller, W. R., & Rollnick, S. (2023). *Motivational interviewing: Helping people change and grow.* Guilford Press.

Singh Ospina, N., Phillips, K. A., Rodriguez-Gutierrez, R., Castaneda-Guarderas, A., Gionfriddo, M. R., Branda, M. E., & Montori, V. M. (2019). Eliciting the patient's agenda—Secondary analysis of recorded clinical encounters. *Journal of General Internal Medicine, 34*(1), 36–40.

SECTION II

Addressing Common Barriers to Rehabilitation Engagement

4   Therapy Participation and Adherence

Kathleen T. Bechtold and Joe Fangman

What Is Rehabilitation Therapy Participation and Adherence?

The rehabilitation process is a series of integrated, therapeutic interventions aimed at improving physical, cognitive, emotional, and life functioning that is shepherded by a wide range of clinicians regardless of the setting. The patient's level of engagement in the rehabilitation process is foundational to the ultimate outcomes that are achieved by each patient across rehabilitation populations (Holliday et al., 2007; Huyser et al., 1997; Kortte et al., 2007; Lenze et al., 2004; Resnick et al., 1998; Skolasky et al., 2008). Thus, ensuring that patients engage fully in the process and adhere to the treatment plan will promote achievement of the best possible outcomes that are meaningful to the patient.

Engagement in rehabilitation has been defined as a deliberate effort and commitment to working toward the goals of rehabilitation interventions, typically demonstrated through active, effortful participation in therapies and cooperation with treatment providers (Lequerica & Kortte, 2010). While rehabilitation participation is a related construct to engagement, it does not necessarily require high levels of invested interest and can be viewed simply as the patient complying or assenting to being treated and being present in the rehabilitation therapy session. Engagement,

Kathleen T. Bechtold and Joe Fangman, *Therapy Participation and Adherence* In: *Motivational Interviewing in Medical Rehabilitation*. Edited by: Nicole Schechter, Connie Jacocks, Lester Butt, and Stephen T. Wegener, Oxford University Press.
© Oxford University Press 2024. DOI: 10.1093/oso/9780197748268.003.0005

on the other hand, can be observed where the person and environment interface and is driven by motivation and executed by the directing of energy and effort toward a therapeutic task or activity. As proposed by Lequerica and Kortte (2010), therapeutic engagement includes two main phases: the motivational phase (i.e., considering engagement in therapy) and the volitional phase (i.e., taking action and reassessing whether to continue engaging). Within the motivational phase, the patient considers the perceived need for treatment (i.e., perception that one has a problem or condition or risk that needs to be addressed to achieve a positive outcome), perceived self-efficacy (i.e., belief about one's abilities with the therapeutic task at hand), and outcome expectancies (i.e., the perception that there will be a successful outcome of value). Once the patient has agreed to engage in the activity (the volitional phase), goal-setting occurs (i.e., preparation to engage); and then, as the patient engages in the therapeutic activity, there is ongoing assessment of the beliefs, attitudes, and expectations (i.e., maintenance of engagement). If the experience is viewed as enjoyable, worthwhile, and/or beneficial, then engagement continues. However, if the experience is seen as pointless, aversive, and/or not helpful or no longer needed, then the patient disengages. As argued by Lequerica and Kortte (2010), understanding the complex process of engagement can assist clinicians in partnering with patients, families, caregivers, and fellow team members to establish meaningful goals, apply effective interventions, and determine appropriate measures of the impact of those interventions.

What Are the Common Challenges to Rehabilitation Therapy Engagement, and Why Do These Matter?

The engagement model can assist in identifying and understanding potential barriers or challenges to the rehabilitation process. Patients do not, at times, consistently show up for rehabilitation therapy activities; and when they do, their level of engagement can be quite variable. Pain, fatigue, mood, and cognitive impairment, among a host of other personal, social, physical, and emotional factors, can affect the level of engagement (e.g., Kringle et al., 2018; Ramanathan-Elion et al., 2016; see also Chapters 8–10). The challenges to treatment adherence and engagement in the therapeutic process may also be presented by caregivers, families, and the treatment team itself (for a more detailed discussion of these challenges, the reader is referred to Chapters 6 and 11). By considering the type of barrier or challenge through the lens of the engagement model, rehabilitation clinicians can tailor the therapeutic interactions and treatment plan development to address many of the treatment challenges that can affect engagement and treatment adherence. Example challenges to therapeutic engagement at different phases of engagement from the viewpoint of the patient, caregiver, family, treatment team, and peer counselor are presented in Table 4.1.

How can rehabilitation clinicians promote their patients engaging in the therapeutic process? It has long been established that the "communicative rapport" between clinicians and patients (Shontz & Fink, 1957) and including them in the decision-making and planning process (Wright, 1960) promote higher levels of engagement. The approach to communication is thus key to truly engaging the patient, family, and fellow team members in the rehabilitation process. In addition, there is evidence that the attitude of the clinician as present, receptive, genuine, and committed affects the therapeutic relationship and thus the engagement of the patient in the therapeutic process (Miciak et al., 2018). These elements that promote therapeutic engagement align extremely well with the motivational interviewing (MI) spirit and skills (Chapters 1 and 3), thus opening a door for rehabilitation clinicians to use MI to promote therapeutic engagement and treatment adherence.

How Can MI Help with Rehabilitation Therapy Engagement Challenges?

MI is all about communication. The MI skills provide guidance to shaping the communication through the types of words chosen and messages conveyed. However, the rehabilitation clinician must keep in mind that the words chosen and messages conveyed are rooted in the attitude of the person shaping that interaction. As discussed in detail in Chapters 1 and 3, the attitude one holds when coming into an interaction and the communication approach taken affect the quality and effectiveness of the interaction. For the rehabilitation clinician to be successful in promoting engagement in the therapeutic process, they need to consider the beliefs and values they bring to the interaction: How do I, as a rehabilitation professional, view the goal of independence? What is my role as a rehabilitation clinician? What is a successful rehabilitation outcome? By considering the foundational principles of MI, the attitude of the clinician is shaped toward a guiding role in which the patient plays a directive role in defining independence and a successful outcome. The four key principles of MI captured by the acronym RULE (Resist the fixing reflex, Understand your client's motives, Listen, and Empower your client) are foundational to the rehabilitation clinician coming to the interaction with the ACE in hand (an attitude of acceptance, compassion, and empowerment) and ready to employ the OARS (open-ended questions, affirmations, reflections, summaries) and tools (asking permission and scaling questions) in order to facilitate the two phases of engagement.

TABLE 4.1

Rehabilitation Therapy Engagement Challenge Examples

	Example challenge	Phase of engagement
Patient	Awareness of deficits: "I just need to rest, and I will get better, then I can get back to home and working."	Perceived need for interventions in motivation phase
	May lead to harm or injury: "I will fall if you make me stand, and then I will be hurt even worse!"	Perceived risk of interventions in motivation phase
Caregiver	Experience is pointless: "If she cannot use the toilet on her own, then what's the use of all of this?"	Analysis of experience in volition phase
	Perceived value of outcome: "You are so focused on him sitting on the edge of the bed. When are you going to get him walking?"	Intention to engage between motivational phase and volitional phase
Family/ support system	Perceived treatment demands: "She cannot talk to me or remember anything. How will she ever be able to do anything for herself?"	Perceived self-efficacy in motivational phase
	Perceived treatment benefits: "I will take care of everything he needs. He does not need to learn about bowel and bladder care."	Perceived need in motivational phase
Treatment team	Setting goals: "This patient is so young. We should make sure she is focusing on returning to work."	Preparation to engage in volitional phase
	Reassessment of beliefs, attitudes, expectations: "This patient is so hard to work with! He expects us to fix him, and he won't listen to what I am telling him to do."	Analysis of experience in volition phase
Peer counseling	Awareness of capabilities: "You have more strength and energy than you give yourself credit for."	Perceived self-efficacy in motivational phase
	Experience is aversive: "The prosthetics hurt me too. You will get over it."	Analysis of experience in volition phase

Being mindful in each interaction of the principles embedded in RULE, described in detail below, helps the rehabilitation clinician maintain a guiding role that truly engages others in the rehabilitation process. Rehabilitation clinicians need to resist the fixing reflex. Many individuals do not respond and engage well when they are told/directed what to do. Clinicians collaborate and guide rather than demand or direct in order to motivate an individual to engage. A rehabilitation nurse coming into a patient's room who has been upset about having to do turns for skin protection could say, "It seems that doing turns is frustrating for you. Is it OK if I share with you how doing turns in bed will help you recover?" This reflection followed by asking permission will go a lot further than coming in and saying, "You need to do a turn or you're going to get a skin sore!" To avoid the fixing reflex, use reflection and summary from the MI skills (OARS) or ask permission to share your expertise.

Rehabilitation clinicians aim to understand the motivation of the other person. The role of a rehabilitation clinician is not to provide motivation for patients but to guide them to discover that motivation for themselves using the MI skills and tools. As the saying goes, "You can lead a horse to water, but you can't make it drink." Evoking questions help clinicians have better understanding of an individual's motivation and readiness for change (and to engage). Evoking questions can include "What are you ready and willing to do?" and "How would you like things to be different?"

Rehabilitation clinicians listen with empathy to step into the other person's shoes. Listening with empathy, a clinician might view the situation from the patient's point of view, understanding their feelings and perspectives toward the treatment being worked on. Employing the MI skills of reflections and summaries supports the rehabilitation clinician in listening with empathy. Rephrase what the patient is telling you using the same elements and wording they used, for example, "You're sharing that you don't feel ready to be doing . . ." Using some reflection and summarizing lets the patient know you are listening and trying to understand their experience and perspective.

Finally, the rehabilitation clinician empowers the patient. This principle gets to the heart of the MI approach and to the motivation phase of engagement. Empowerment is rooted in the patient perceiving the need for treatment, believing in their ability to engage in the task or activity at hand (i.e., self-efficacy), and expecting that these efforts will be successful, helpful, and/or meaningful. Using the MI skills of affirming, reflecting, and asking open-ended questions empowers the patient to find the value in the treatment and the confidence in their ability to engage and that engagement will lead to outcomes that they will find meaningful.

To further assist rehabilitation clinicians in maintaining their ACE throughout an interaction, the MI tool of asking permission is employed. Rather than telling the patient "I am going to show you how to . . . [e.g., position yourself so you do not get a skin breakdown]," try asking "Is it OK if I share some techniques on how to . . . [e.g., position yourself so you do not get skin breakdown]?" By asking permission and getting an affirmative, the rehabilitation clinician has invited the patient, family member, or caregiver to take an active role in the therapy and engage more fully in the process.

Asking scaling questions is another MI tool that helps to gauge an individual's confidence in a skill or the importance of a skill or activity when setting goals and priorities for treatment progression. Asking a patient, "On a scale of 1 to 10, where 1 is not important and 10 is very important, how would you rate [transfers, getting back to work, self-care, decreasing your pain, etc.]?" If the individual gives a rating of 6, the rehabilitation clinician could comment "That's most interesting. How come it's not a 4?" or could use a follow-up question, "What activities would you rate as a 10?" This is a great way to set meaningful goals and priorities with the patient understanding their motivation and empowering them to engage in the treatments.

The use of scaling questions can also be very beneficial in assessing a patient's confidence with a skill. Asking a patient "On a scale of 1 to 10, where 1 is not confident and 10 is extremely confident, how would you rate your confidence in your ability to [transfer from wheelchair to supine in bed, catheterize yourself, don and doff your prosthetic, etc.]?" Then the rehabilitation clinician can follow up that question with the question "How can we work together to go from a 6 to an 8?" Scaling offers a tangible way for patients to visualize their thoughts about a task or activity and convey that level of importance and confidence to the rehabilitation clinician. Table 4.2 provides examples of challenging situations that can be encountered by rehabilitation clinicians and example statements using MI skills (OARS) and tools to respond to the challenge with the goal of facilitating therapeutic engagement.

Although it is recognized that coming to an interaction with another person with the RULE in mind and the ACE up the sleeve will facilitate that interaction, each element of the MI spirit can weigh more heavily depending on the context and content of that interaction. Similarly, relying upon the entire OARS throughout an interaction will result in a more productive and successful interaction, but within the interaction, the context and content may pull for one or another of the MI skills. Table 4.3 is a summary of the phases of therapeutic engagement mapped with the MI spirit, skills, and tools to highlight the alignment. For each element within the two phases of the engagement process, the particular attitude (spirit), skill, or tool to keep in mind is noted.

TABLE 4.2

Using Your OARS: Example Questions and Statements to Facilitate Therapeutic Engagement and Adherence

Situation	OARS
Patient/client frustrated with a therapeutic session	"How do you think we can work together more constructively?" (Open-ended question)
Patient/client not liking the direction of the program or treatment	"What are your main goals so we can make sure we are heading in the same direction?" (Open-ended question)
Patient/client frustrated with another discipline wanting them to do more for themselves and telling you what that discipline wants them to do	"It seems that you don't feel ready to ... [e.g., manage own continence, transfer, learn own meds, perform self-care]. Tell me more." (Reflection/Open-ended question)
Patient/client reporting how they cannot be independent and must rely on family for help and being frustrated with what the future holds and not being a burden to their family	"It sounds like family is important to you and you want to provide for them and not burden them." (Reflection)
Patient/client not following through on home exercise program	"Help me understand how the home exercise program is difficult for you." (Open-ended question)
Patient/client not wanting to continue therapy because they are not seeing progress even with effort	"What is missing from your therapy program?" (Open-ended question)
Patient/client being ambivalent about discharge	"What are your top concerns before discharge" (Open-ended questions)
Patient/client starting to have self-doubt about progress in therapy after working so hard for past few weeks	"You have persevered through so much." "You have been working very hard at ... [learning about self-cathing, working on transfers]." (Affirmation)
Patient/client discussing frustration with discharge options and talking with clinician	"So what I am hearing from you is. ... What did I miss?" (Summary/Open-ended question)

Note. OARS = open-ended questions, affirmations, reflections, summaries.

TABLE 4.3

Parallels Between the Elements of Therapeutic Engagement and Motivational Interviewing

Elements of therapeutic engagement			Motivational interviewing	
			Spirit	Skills and tools
Motivational phase				
Perceived need	The belief that there is a deficit or simply room for improvement to reach a desired goal coupled with the belief	Awareness of deficits	Acceptance Compassion Partnership	Open-ended questions Affirmation Asking permission
	that the involvement in the treatment or activity will reduce this deficit or risk or help achieve the desired goal	Perceived treatment benefits	Empowerment/ understanding partnership	Open-ended questions Affirmations Reflections Asking permission
Perceived risk	The perception of risk associated with the therapeutic activity coupled with the value of	May lead to harm or injury (e.g., fear of falling)	Compassion Empowerment/ understanding partnership	Open-ended questions Reflections
	the outcome and/or belief of likelihood of success despite the risk	May be unpleasant process (e.g., increased pain)	Compassion Empowerment/ understanding partnership	Open-ended questions Reflections
Perceived self-efficacy	The belief in one's capacity to meet the demands of treatment coupled with the value of the outcome and/or belief of likelihood of success	Awareness of capabilities	Compassion Empowerment/ understanding partnership	Open-ended questions Affirmations Reflections
		Perceived treatment demands	Empowerment/ understanding partnership	Open-ended questions Reflections
Volitional phase				
Preparation for engagement	Treatment planning occurs by setting goals	Meaning and importance of the goals	Empowerment/ understanding partnership	Open-ended questions Readiness ruler Summary Scaling

TABLE 4.3 *Continued*

Elements of therapeutic engagement			Motivational interviewing	
			Spirit	Skills and tools
Maintenance of engagement	Experience of enjoyment or meaningfulness during therapeutic process versus experience that therapeutic activity is pointless/ unachievable or aversive	Analysis of the experience	Acceptance Compassion Empowerment/ understanding partnership	Open-ended questions Affirmations Reflections Summary Scaling

Note: Adapted from Lequerica and Kortte (2010).

Case Examples

The following case examples, along with the videos available at https://www.reha bengage.org/, demonstrate the use of MI skills and tools to promote therapeutic engagement.

CASE 1

Charlie is a 42-year-old man who sustained a C6 American Spinal Injury Association Impairment Scale C motor incomplete spinal cord injury when he dove too deep into the shallow end of a swimming pool. He has been a patient in the inpatient rehabilitation program for the past 6 weeks. He has good strength in biceps and wrist extensors, fair strength in both triceps, and trace quads and adductors bilaterally in his lower extremities. Charlie is a successful teacher and coach, father to an 8-year-old son, and husband of 10 years. He has been very determined to get better with his main goals of "walking and being normal again" and does not want his wife helping him with any of his self-care or daily life functioning. Charlie rarely smiles, does not want his wife posting anything about his injury on social media, and emotionally breaks down during sessions on a weekly basis. He works hard and often cusses and gets angry with himself in therapy. Charlie has been attending all therapy sessions and reminds therapists daily that his goal is to walk. His greatest struggle is with completing self-care, particularly learning to complete his own bowel program and self-catheterization. He allows the nurse to complete any bowel care and catheterization but covers his head during these activities and refuses to attempt any of the steps for himself. He is 3 weeks from discharge, and his treatment team knows he has the physical and cognitive ability to do self-catheterization for bladder management and independent bowel management. His physical therapist (PT) has established a good rapport with him and is working with him in his room on transfers.

> PT: "You are working really hard on these transfers today. You really are committed to getting stronger." (Affirmation)
>
> CHARLIE: "Yeah, I want to be back to doing everything on my own, but getting to that wheelchair is not walking!"
>
> PT2: "True, walking is your overall goal, and it sounds like you want to be self-reliant too. Help me to understand what other concerns or goals you have as we work toward you feeling ready to go home?" (Summary, Open-ended question)
>
> CHARLIE: "Walking is the big goal. I won't consider anything less than that a success, but I would like to be able to do stuff for myself and be able to throw a football with my son."
>
> PT: "While walking is your ultimate goal, you're able to appreciate that other goals are also worthwhile. What kind of stuff do you want to be able to do for yourself?" (Reflection, Open-ended question)
>
> CHARLIE: "You know, like get in and out of bed by myself, go to the bathroom by myself, not have a bowel accident every day. I cannot stand having the nurse cath me. I cannot even watch, and the thought of doing it myself, oh I can't even."
>
> PT: "So what I hear you saying is you want to be able to do more for yourself and not rely on others, and cathing sounds like it is tough to wrap your head around." (Summary)
>
> CHARLIE: "Yeah, and there is no way I want my wife to clean me up after a bowel accident or to have to insert the catheter for me."
>
> PT: "Being self-reliant is important to you. It also sounds like you want your wife to be your wife and not have to be a nurse for you. Tell me what you know about self-catheterization, and then you can tell me what steps of self-catheterization you are open to trying." (Affirmation, Open-ended question)
>
> CHARLIE: "Oh. I know all the steps. I pay attention when the nurses tell me, and I have even written them down. I just can't watch them doing it, and I don't think I could do it myself."
>
> PT: "You are resourceful, and you are persevering through learning a lot. Writing down the steps has helped you learn how to self-cath, and trying those steps right now seems like a lot to take on. Is it OK if I share a couple other suggestions with you?" (Affirmation, Reflection, Asking permission)
>
> CHARLIE: "Yes."

PT: "You said doing all the steps right now is not happening. What about breaking down the whole process into smaller, manageable steps? What steps do you think you could work on tonight?" (Summary, Open-ended question)

CHARLIE: "Well, maybe cleaning before inserting the catheter and then just watching the nurse."

PT: "Awesome! It sounds like tonight you are going to do the prep to stay clean during a cath and then watch what the nurse does to help you cath. Let me know how it goes tomorrow." (Summary)

CHARLIE: "OK."

NEXT DAY

PT: "So how did the cathing go last night?" (Open-ended question)

CHARLIE: "I did it, wasn't easy, but I did it."

PT: "Sounds like you gained some confidence. On a scale from 1 to 10, how confident are you that you can do the entire process?" (Reflection, Scaling question)

CHARLIE: "I think a 4."

PT: "A 4 . . . how come not a 2?" (Open-ended question)

CHARLIE: "I realized that there was a lot I already knew, and after doing it once, I know I can do it."

PT: "What would get you to a 6?" (Open-ended question)

CHARLIE: "I think just more time to practice and working with OT [occupational therapy] to make sure that my technique is good. I am sure I can do this. I just need to get over my fear of inserting the catheter myself."

CASE 2

Taylor is a 24-year-old woman who was involved in a motor vehicle collision and sustained multiple traumatic injuries to her lower extremities. After numerous surgeries, she required bilateral below-the-knee amputations. She is currently in an inpatient rehab program. Before her injuries, Taylor was an active 24-year-old who liked to do triathlons with her running group and enjoyed going to clubs and dancing with friends. She is experiencing significant phantom limb and residual limb pain. Although she sometimes goes to therapy, there have been several days this week when she refused to get out of bed to attend her rehab therapy sessions. She states that her goal is to walk and run again. When the nurses crack the door to come into her room and ask her "Are you ready to get up?," she throws a pillow at the wall and yells "No, leave me alone." Taylor has refused to interact with many on the nursing staff. A new nurse who just got back from an MI boot camp and just read this book is working with Taylor today.

NURSE: "Good morning, Taylor. Is it OK if I come in?" (Asking permission)

TAYLOR: "I guess."

NURSE: "My name is Jason. I am a new nurse on the floor. It's nice to meet you. How was your night?" (Open-ended question)

TAYLOR: "I couldn't sleep at all. This dang pain where my right foot was and the end of my stump on the left burned all night. When it hurts like this, I don't get sleep and I just want to cover up and never get out of bed."

NURSE: "Sounds like you had a tough night with the pain. What has helped when you have had this pain in the past week?" (Reflection, Open-ended question)

TAYLOR: "The medications help some, but I don't want to get addicted to those. I have too many other things I want to do and can't be getting hooked on medications. I am fearful of getting addicted to the meds."

NURSE: "You know yourself and know you don't want to become reliant on the meds. If the pain was better managed, what types of activities do you want to be able to do?" (Affirmation, Reflection, Open-ended question)

I want to get back to doing what I love to do."

NURSE: "You mentioned running . . . in what kind of running were you involved?" (Open-ended question)

TAYLOR: "I was doing two to three triathlons a year and going out with friends to clubs on most weekends to dance. I also just landed my dream job. I want to get back to all of that. This injury is not going to stop me."

NURSE: "You are ambitious, motivated, and ready to get back to your life. It seems that if your pain was better controlled, you would be ready take on everything ahead." (Affirmation, Reflection)

TAYLOR: "I sure would."

NURSE: "Would it be OK if I give you your meds and then come back in 15 minutes to help get you up and ready for your day?" (Asking permission)

TAYLOR: "Yes, hopefully in 15 minutes the pain is better. Can we also talk about how I can keep from getting addicted to the pain meds. I want to use them because they help me to do the therapy, but I don't want to become reliant on them."

NURSE: "Sounds like you care about your body and your health. If you had more information about how to use the medication as one tool in your toolkit to help you manage the pain and not become reliant on it, you would be open to using this tool. I can come back this afternoon when you have a break, and we can talk about your medications and how the entire team can help you to use your tools and reach your goals." (Reflection, Summary)

Summary

Rehabilitation professionals shepherd patients through the therapeutic process with the goal of improving physical, cognitive, emotional, and life functioning. Ensuring that patients engage fully in the therapy tasks and activities and adhere to the treatment plan leads to the accomplishment of that goal. Therapeutic engagement is a multiphase process that when understood can help rehabilitation clinicians to tailor the therapeutic interactions and treatment plan to address many of the treatment challenges that can affect engagement and treatment adherence. Additionally, rehabilitation professionals can promote therapeutic engagement and treatment adherence through applying the MI spirit and skills during interactions. Through this approach to communication, patients, family members, and fellow team members can be guided to truly engage in the rehabilitation process, resulting in the best possible outcomes that are meaningful to the patient.

References

Holliday, R. C., Ballinger, C., & Playford, E. D. (2007). Goal setting in neurological rehabilitation: Patients' perspectives. *Disability Rehabilitation, 29*(5), 389–394.

Huyser, B., Buckelew, S. P., Hewett, J. E., & Johnson, J. C. (1997). Factors affecting adherence to rehabilitation interventions for individuals with fibromyalgia. *Rehabilitation Psychology, 42*, 75–91.

Kortte, K. B., Falk, L. D., Castillo, R. C., Johnson-Greene, D., & Wegener, S. T. (2007). The Hopkins Rehabilitation Engagement Rating Scale: Development and psychometric properties. *Archives of Physical Medicine & Rehabilitation, 88*(7), 877–884.

Kringle, E. A., Terhorst, L., Butters, M. A., & Skidmore, E. R. (2018). Clinical predictors of engagement in inpatient rehabilitation among stroke survivors with cognitive deficits: An exploratory study. *Journal of the International Neuropsychological Society, 24*(6), 572–583.

Lenze, E. J., Munin, M. C., Dew, M. A., Rogers, J. C., Seligman, K., Mulsant, B. H., & Reynolds, C. F., 3rd. (2004). Adverse effects of depression and cognitive impairment on rehabilitation participation and recovery from hip fracture. *International Journal of Geriatric Psychiatry, 19*, 472–478.

Lequerica, A. H., & Kortte, K. B. (2010). Therapeutic engagement: A proposed model of engagement in medical rehabilitation. *American Journal of Physical Medicine & Rehabilitation, 89*(5), 415–422.

Miciak, M., Mayan, M., Brown, C., Joyce, A. S., & Gross, D. P. (2018). The necessary conditions of engagement for the therapeutic relationship in physiotherapy: An interpretive description study. *Archives of Physiotherapy, 8*(3), Article 3. https://doi.org/10.1186/s40945-018-0044-1

Ramanathan-Elion, D., McWhorter, J., Wegener, S. T., & Bechtold, K. T. (2016). The role of psychological facilitators and barriers to therapeutic engagement in acute, inpatient rehabilitation. *Rehabilitation Psychology*, *61*, 277–287.

Resnick, B., Zimmerman, S., Magaziner, J., & Adelman, A. (1998). Use of the Apathy Evaluation Scale as a measure of motivation in elderly people. *Rehabilitation Nursing*, *23*, 141–147.

Shontz, F. C., & Fink, S. L. (1957). The significance of patient–staff rapport in the rehabilitation of individuals with chronic physical illness. *Journal of Consulting Psychology*, *21*(4), 327–334.

Skolasky, R. L., Mackenzie, E. J., Wegener, S. T., & Riley, L. H., III. (2008). Patient activation and adherence to physical therapy in persons undergoing spine surgery. *Spine*, *33*, E784–E791.

Wright, B. (1960). *Physical disability: A psychological approach*. Harper & Row Publishers.

5   Self-Management
Danbi Lee, Maureen Gecht-Silver, and Linda Ehrlich-Jones

What Is Self-Management?

Self-management includes tasks such as medical, emotional, and role management that individuals must undertake to live with one or more chronic conditions. It is an approach that allows patients to build skills, knowledge, and
confidence in managing their medical conditions and achieve an impact on their
everyday life. Self-management is a dynamic and continuous process of negotiating the impact of chronic conditions on physical, emotional, and social parts of
everyday life.

Rehabilitation professionals can provide self-management support to enhance
patient activation and self-management. The goal of self-management support
is to share information and teach self-management skills and techniques by providing patients with opportunities to build self-efficacy and autonomy so that
they feel confident managing their life with chronic conditions. Essential components for facilitating a patient's development of self-management skills include
patient education, support for lifestyle modifications, and support to help
individuals develop the knowledge and skills needed for effective chronic disease management (e.g., negotiating behavior changes through problem-solving,

Danbi Lee, Maureen Gecht-Silver, and Linda Ehrlich-Jones, *Self-Management* In: *Motivational Interviewing in Medical Rehabilitation.*
Edited by: Nicole Schechter, Connie Jacocks, Lester Butt, and Stephen T. Wegener, Oxford University Press.
© Oxford University Press 2024. DOI: 10.1093/oso/9780197748268.003.0006

action-planning, and goal setting; Barlow et al., 2002; Centers for Disease Control and Prevention, 2020).

What Are the Challenges to Engagement in Self-Management?

Integrating self-management support into rehabilitation and engaging patients in self-management can be challenging. Rehabilitation provides services to a wide range of people and conditions (from hip fracture to Parkinson's disease) in a variety of settings (e.g., inpatient, outpatient, community). People who have lived with disabilities or chronic conditions for a while are more likely to be experts on their health and have routines that work for them. Many have learned to listen to their body and know when to rest or seek healthcare. When conditions change, what the patient chooses to do may not be aligned with the clinician's preferences. If the clinician maintains the expert role by only telling the patient what to do or assuming that the clinician's perspective is the only correct one, it may be difficult to promote patient partnership and autonomy. On the other hand, people who just acquired new impairments lack the awareness and experience of living with a disability at home and in the community without professional help. It may be hard for them to imagine and prepare for life after discharge. Because self-management is typically a skill that patients learn and start using once they are home from rehabilitation, engaging patients in conversations about self-management early on can be tricky.

There are a number of challenges to patient engagement in self-management especially in inpatient rehabilitation. First, patients are often tired from therapies and overwhelmed with the changes to their body and perhaps their entire life. Second, there is uncertainty with what their life will look like, and often there is a strong desire to completely regain functions that would allow them to go back to their previous life. Not all patients will appreciate being reminded that their life will likely be different and have challenging aspects when they leave the hospital. Third, when patients have a goal that is different from a clinician's or have a goal that a clinician might think they are not ready for yet, there can be tension between the clinician and patient. When there is no acceptance or respect for the patient as an expert in their life, this tension and power struggle can hinder clinicians from building true partnership with them and engaging them. This struggle, whether it is noticeable or subtle, is common when clinicians have their own agenda based on outcomes expected by the system (frequently, improving function related to patients' safety) and push patients to accomplish them.

While self-management support is the process of teaching patients skills of self-management such as problem-solving, decision-making, action-planning, finding and using resources, communication, and self- monitoring, it cannot be achieved without partnering and sharing the power. When patients continue to see health-care professionals as experts with all the answers, it is less likely that they will be confident in making decisions around their healthcare. Clinicians need to give space for patients to see themselves as the agent of their life and feel empowered to use self-management skills to make important decisions. This can only be achieved when clinicians temper the expert role and put more emphasis on collaborating with patients. Motivational interviewing (MI) provides clinicians with a patient-centered communication approach that can facilitate the process of building self-management in a collaborative way.

Why Do These Challenges Matter?

There is increasing evidence that effective self-management is essential to optimiz-ing health outcomes for people with chronic conditions. While self-management has been historically used to support people with chronic conditions such as diabe-tes, asthma, and arthritis, it also has an important role in the context of rehabilita-tion conditions such as stroke, brain injury, or spinal cord injury. After injuries or onsets of life-changing medical conditions, people frequently experience health and functional problems (e.g., paralysis/weakness, pain, fatigue, cognitive impairment), activity and participation restrictions, and environmental barriers (e.g., trouble get-ting in the car, difficulty visiting friends due to inaccessible buildings, trouble going out when snowing or due to financial hardship). To address these long lasting effects, there is a need for understanding these acute events as chronic conditions and pro-viding services that align with chronic care principles (Jones et al., 2013).

While functional recovery of neurological functioning and self-care capability is an important rehabilitation outcome for people with conditions such as stroke, brain injury, or spinal cord injury, it may not be sufficient to help them rebuild their lives. Self-management skills can help patients identify strategies to address medical and emotional needs and changes in their roles and lives.

MEDICAL MANAGEMENT

Medical management involves tasks such as following through on treatments and healthy behaviors (e.g., doing exercises, eating well, taking medications, using equipment as advised), monitoring and noticing symptoms (e.g., fatigue, pain) and changes in health, and making decisions on how to respond to symptoms or changes with or without professional help. Some patients in rehabilitation develop greater interest in healthy behaviors as a means to recover and prevent secondary conditions or because they believe poor health behaviors contributed to their medical event. Improved medical management is associated with positive outcomes such as decreased rehospitalization and decreased morbidity and mortality (Afshin et al., 2019; Billinger et al., 2014; Ruppar et al., 2016).

A common mistake clinicians make is to blame or judge patients for being "nonadherent" or "noncompliant" with medical management directives. For example, medication management may be a challenge when patients do not have knowledge of their medications, prefer not taking certain medications, fear side effects, have cognitive impairment hindering management, do not have a good relationship with the provider, or lack proper access to healthcare (Guilcher et al., 2019). Similarly, barriers to exercising or being physically active may be internal, such as low motivation or confidence, and limited skills, or external, such as an unsafe neighborhood, stigma toward people with disabilities, or lack of access to reliable and affordable transportation or accessible gyms (Rimmer et al., 2004; Scelza et al., 2005). When it comes to healthy eating, many people know what they should and should not eat and drink; research shows that common barriers to healthy eating is often not patients' knowledge but rather access to healthy food or other external factors (Clifford & Curtis, 2015). As such, it is a clinician's responsibility to facilitate collaborative problem-solving and goal-setting, which involves identifying these underlying obstacles. Doing so requires clinicians to build partnership and trust with patients.

EMOTIONAL MANAGEMENT

Emotional management involves noticing and finding ways to manage common emotional impacts of having a chronic condition such as fear, anger, uncertainty, despair, frustration, anxiety, and depression. While many patients experience emotional difficulties, emotional management is often not addressed in rehabilitation, and patients have identified emotional support as an unmet need (Bamm et al., 2015; Loft et al., 2019; Peoples et al., 2011). Acquiring new medical conditions and/ or chronic impairments is often a life-changing experience that comes with worries, uncertainty, and anxiety. It is not a surprise that many patients are depressed and overwhelmed with thoughts about the future and desire to talk about those thoughts and concerns (Loft et al., 2019). Studies have pointed out depression as a predictor of decreased social participation and life satisfaction (Ezekiel et al., 2019), supporting the importance of addressing emotions during rehabilitation. Promoting development of coping strategies as part of rehabilitation would provide opportunities to assess feelings, needs, and self-management strategies to apply to future situations and promote long-term acceptance of their new self. Self-management support for emotion management can be addressed in an interdisciplinary way where emotions are talked about within different contexts by different team members. Depending on the clinical focus, clinicians can address emotions around role changes, pain, health-related uncertainty, medications, or walking capacity as they support the person with goals in these areas.

ROLE MANAGEMENT

Role management involves maintaining, changing, and developing meaningful life roles while managing the impact of the chronic conditions and their interaction with the environment. People come to rehabilitation with a history of life roles as partners, parents, workers, caregivers, and more. These roles give their life meaning and purpose. People have the desire to continue their previous roles or develop new ones. However, finding ways of engaging in roles and activities after an injury, onset of disease, or exacerbation can be difficult. People living with chronic conditions or chronic impairments report higher rates of decreased engagement in life activities and dissatisfaction with life involvement (Ginis et al., 2021; Palstam et al., 2019). Participation in life roles is critical and has important health implications. Research has consistently shown that unsatisfactory participation in meaningful activities and roles and social isolation have negative impacts on physical and emotional health, well-being, and quality of life (Algurén et al., 2012; Ang, 2019; Feng et al., 2020).

Like medical management, managing roles and life activities can be a complex process and requires strategies on multiple levels. Clinicians can begin this process during rehabilitation by helping people gain comfort with asking for help, engaging them in problem-solving related to their specific concerns, setting action plans to practice and gain confidence, and exploring creative ways to adapt activities and the environment and relearn specific skills. It can go as far as providing information so that patients understand their rights and gain confidence in asking for accommodations and resources and advocating for systemic changes that may be necessary to participate fully in society. Collaborating with people in rehabilitation to prioritize meaningful roles and identify small steps to reintegrate these tasks and roles is critical to confidence-building. While it can be challenging for patients to identify potential barriers to re-engaging in previous roles and find solutions while in the hospital, rehabilitation is an important place to initiate this conversation so that they become accustomed to the process while they have professional support. Using MI gives clinicians a framework to engage patients in these types of conversations and evoke their motivation to plan ahead with self-identified problems and solutions.

How Can MI Support Engagement in Self-Management?

MI skills are critical to building motivation and partnership. MI can also facilitate self-management readiness by evoking the patient's treatment priorities, values, and meaningful activities they aspire to return to. Actively engaging patients in activities they enjoy, such as hobbies, can inspire curiosity, problem-solving, and development of a realistic plan for determining adaptations and assistance needed. MI skills can be useful to address ambivalence and overcome frustrations as they arise.

Although the need for self-management in patients' post-rehabilitation life and thus the need for self-management support during rehabilitation is evident, it is not always clear what steps clinicians can take to enhance patient self-management. The 12 evidence-based principles for implementing self-management support by Battersby et al. (2010) highlight the importance of shared decision-making, collaborative goal-setting, problem-solving, and nonjudgmental attitude by clinicians as critical components that make self-management support effective. MI provides a set of skills and principles that can guide clinicians to share power with their patients and create nonjudgmental, strength-based communication that promotes self-management.

When clinicians enlist the patient's expertise about their life and valued activities, opportunities for tailoring therapy to their life emerge. The therapist can develop this further through inclusion of practice in self-monitoring, identifying issues, prioritizing, and engaging patients in problem-solving and decision-making. In an inpatient setting, instead of telling step by step what to do for tub transfer, therapists can use MI and self-management support by giving the patient a chance to try the activity, observe and describe what they can or cannot do, brainstorm different ways of doing it, and make decisions and plans collaboratively. MI spirit and skills can ensure that the process of building patient self-management is more patient-centered, contextualizes and prioritizes problems important to patients, and evokes patients' motivation while focusing on patients' strengths, values, and change talk. Table 5.1 summarizes key principles for self-management support and how those principles can be achieved in an MI-consistent manner. While MI spirit and skills can be used with any of these principles, the table highlights key strategies that would ensure self-management support is offered in an MI-consistent way.

TABLE 5.1

MI-Consistent Implementation of Self-Management Support Principles

Principles	Description	MI-consistent manner
Shared decision-making	• Avoid providing information only • Discussion between the patient and clinician to determine interventions appropriate for the patient.	• Ask for permission • Partner with the patient • Ask-offer-Ask to identify what they want to know • Clinician and patient share and discuss ideas about their decision
Collaborative goal-setting	• Patient and clinician work together to define the problem and set a realistic goal	• Determine patient strength • Have patients identify areas they want to work on • Use bubble chart for broader options • Elicit and cultivate change talk • Help patients prioritize and add input for patient to consider
Collaborative problem-solving	• Patient and clinician work together to define a problem, brainstorm possible solutions, choose a strategy, try it, evaluate the outcome, and repeat the process	• Use nonjudgmental attitude and listen to patient's ideas • Help patients prioritize an area to work on and an idea to try out • Help patient identify their strengths that will help them move forward, not just problems • As needed, reflect back and summarize • Offer suggestions only after drawing out the patient's ideas
Active follow-up	• Clinician provides active follow-up including feedback and reminders to help sustain behavior changes	• Ask for permission • Engage with patients to explore what has and has not been going well • Check in to promote accountability to help patients identify future directions

Note: MI = motivational interviewing.

Examples of how MI can support self-management will be presented in the next section with two short case scenarios and scripts.

MI Spirit, Tasks, and Skills

MI offers clinicians a framework to build a collaborative relationship with patients, creating room for patients to share their goals and participate in their own treatment. This collaborative and person-centered conversation style can facilitate the resolution of ambivalence, elicit motivation and commitment for behavior change, and promote patients' active role in assuming responsibility for their life and care. The following section outlines how components of MI can complement the process of self-management support.

MI SPIRIT

MI spirit involves partnership, acceptance, empowerment, and compassion, which create a framework for the attitude of the clinician. (For more detail, see Chapter 1.) When clinicians incorporate MI spirit, patients will feel more involved and in control, which is a first important step toward self-management. In an effort to show respect and share power (partnership), clinicians can get into a habit of asking for permission such as before providing information. Showing patients respect and listening with a nonjudgmental open mind builds trust and engagement with them (acceptance), which sets the stage for more effective problem-solving, decision-making, and goal-setting. Empowerment reminds the clinician that the patient's values and motivation drive change and that self-management ultimately is carried out by the patient. When the patient is ambivalent about making changes or putting out effort, MI can help the patient build reasons to engage in self-management or work through current or potential problems and make plans and changes with clinicians. Sometimes the desired direction of the patient and the clinician will not match. This can be a challenge especially for the health professional who is working in a system that may not have the same priorities as the patient. When a strong relationship is developed between the provider and the patient, this can be easier to work through. When compassion for the patient evokes a warm-hearted feeling, it can inspire the clinician to help the patient progress. Compassion allows clinicians to step back and understand the patient's perspective and look out for their welfare. It can also soften frustration and judgment toward patients not progressing quickly or struggling. The clinician's belief in the potential of the patient to progress can influence patient outcomes, and when the beliefs are positive it can hold the hope until the client has their own (Miller & Moyers, 2021).

MI TASKS

The four MI processes or tasks, give clinicians a guide and remind them about the importance of engaging first and then focusing and evoking so that patients build their own motivation that will take them to planning. (For more detail, see Chapter 3.) Therapeutic engagement is a prerequisite to any self-management support activities. By engaging, focusing, and evoking, clinicians can better understand their patients, build partnerships and alliances, and identify target behaviors that are important to patients. This task allows clinicians and patients to be on the same page and see each other as partners as they set self-management goals and work together in treatment sessions. It can also support patients' autonomy and resolve ambivalence. When the patient builds their own motivation, it can lead them to plan, problem-solve, and make decisions with hope and confidence.

Like any intervention, the four tasks are not linear. When patients experience setbacks or changes in their status, clinicians need to re-engage with patients or evoke their motivation again. It is important to not engage patients in planning before they build motivation and readiness as it can lead to premature action-planning and lower likelihood of making changes (Miller & Rollnick, 2013, 2023). When clinicians are not sure where to go next in supporting patient self-management, reviewing MI tasks can help assess and provide direction. Some questions that clinicians can ask themselves include the following: Did I engage the person? Were there too many ideas? Was the conversation focused? Did the person set a goal that they are truly interested in working on? Did I pressure the patient to make choices? Are there other things (e.g., social determinants of health) that are preventing this person from achieving what they want? Did I take the time to understand this person's perspective? With these self-directed questions, clinicians may be able to find the missing brick and revisit the MI process that can support the foundation for moving forward with self-management support.

MI SKILLS

Open-ended questions, affirmation, reflective listening, summarizing, and information exchange are useful skills to integrate into self-management support to help explore concerns and elicit conversations about change. (For more detail, see Chapter 3.) Open-ended questions are exploratory and evocative questions that can make patients think about the importance of making changes and prioritize based on their values and strengths. First, open-ended questions allow clinicians to identify where to intervene. For example, for medication management, open-ended questions will allow the patient to discuss what issues are of concern with their medication management and identify where they need help. Evocative open-ended questions often elicit change talk, which can positively impact self-management support. Self-management support focuses on finding strategies to address identified barriers and problems. Open-ended questions in MI can be used to go beyond sustain talk and focus on how to overcome barriers, rather than expanding on identified barriers, to help patients talk themselves into change. When patients talk about barriers, they are reinforcing the idea that there are reasons they cannot self-manage. Clinicians can change the course of the conversation by asking evocative questions that elicit possibilities of overcoming barriers. For example, when a patient who recently fell does not want to use a walker, a physical therapist can ask the patient questions such as What concerns do you have about your recent fall? How do you feel about your recent fall? What benefits do you see to using your walker more regularly? or If you were going to use the walker more often, how would you go about that? When patients have difficulty identifying strategies for making changes, clinicians may ask what past successes the patient had with dealing with similar situations. Such probes can help patients to find their own ways to create new habits or address barriers that are more likely to be successful.

Affirmation acknowledges patients' strengths and positive actions and behaviors, which is different from praising. Self-management support aims to provide opportunities that will improve patients' confidence in engaging in self-management tasks; however, it is not always feasible to engage patients in self-management tasks in a hospital setting. Affirmation offers a tool to support patients' self-efficacy in any context. For example, a speech–language pathologist working with a patient with aphasia may use affirmation by saying "You were able to take your time and share your ideas without getting frustrated. I noticed a few rest breaks really helped you," instead of "You did a good job today." Affirmation can instill patient self-efficacy and motivation to want to do more that may give patients a positive outlook.

Reflective listening builds trust and mutual understanding and promotes a non-judgmental attitude. It lays the foundation for collaborative self-management support. It can be a helpful tool in engaging in conversations around sensitive and difficult topics such as emotions or concerns about the future. By making the best guess at what the person means, reflection can make patients feel heard and understood, which then leads to trust. With reflections, clinicians can also help patients better understand their own views or situation, which may raise their self-awareness of where self-management is needed and motivate them to make changes. When used in a forward-moving and evocative way, it can help patients focus on their priorities and increase their desire to engage in self-management. For example, an occupational therapist (OT) may use reflections to help a patient gain greater understanding of their situation and focus on what is most important to them.

PATIENT: "My family is the only comfort right now, and I worry about being a burden to them."

OT: "It's very important for you to find ways to regain your independence."

PATIENT: "Yes, that is really important to me. My first priority is finding out how much I can do at home."

OT: "You want to figure out what you can and cannot do."

Summarizing is a special form of reflective listening that acknowledges patients' ambivalence and change talk. Summarizing often ends with a question to assist in putting it together or eliciting next steps. Clinicians can use summarizing selectively and strategically to recognize ambivalence and gather and share change talk to promote self-management. It can be used during a conversation to refocus the conversation and/or at the end to recap what the clinician observed and heard with a chance to use that information to plan about the next step. For example, a physical therapist may end a home health session on exercising with a summary:

"Part of you doesn't like doing the exercises. But when you do them, you feel better. You found that it is the easiest when you do them right out of bed in the morning, and taking a break in between exercises makes it more doable and you are less tired. Today, you were able to do all the exercises accurately. Where would you like to go from here?"

Information exchange (ask-offer-ask) is another important skill. Patients may have incorrect information or not have the information they want and need to self-manage. It has been the tendency of clinicians to give that information in a directive and nontailored manner. The process of ask–offer–ask allows the clinician to figure out what information the patient needs; provide small, manageable amounts of information; and then talk with the patient about their reaction to the information, how they will use it, or if they understand what was expressed. When information or professional opinion needs to be offered, ask for permission. A nurse might provide medication education using the ask-offer-ask approach.

NURSE: "What do you understand about the reasons for taking each of your medications?" (Ask)

PATIENT: "I know this one is to keep my blood pressure under control. What is this one? Warfarin?"

NURSE: "Yes. Would you like to know what the other medication is and what it does?" (Ask)

PATIENT: "Sure. My pharmacist told me what it is, and I forgot. That is also the one that I sometimes forget to take on time."

NURSE: "Warfarin is a blood thinner. If blood sticks together to form clots, they can travel to your brain and cause another stroke. Warfarin keeps clots from getting bigger and moving to another part of the body. This helps the body system to break down a clot over time and reduces the chance of clots developing in people with a higher risk of forming clots." (Offer) "What do you make of this?" (Ask)

PATIENT: "Wow. That sounds important. I should make more effort to take it as prescribed."

Table 5.2 shows specific examples of how MI can be used in self-management support by different disciplines. The examples focus on using MI to promote the role management of a 53-year-old woman with multiple sclerosis who is currently in relapse and seen in outpatient rehabilitation. The person wants to resume her professional role as an artist. She is hoping to attend an annual social event for local artists to stay in touch with her professional network but feels uneasy about the idea.

Case Studies

Here are two case studies which highlight how MI skills can be used in self-management support in rehabilitation.

CASE 1

Sarah is a 60-year-old woman with a history of osteoarthritis. She had an elective surgery of a total hip replacement due to increasing pain. After the surgery and a short hospitalization, she was transferred to subacute inpatient rehabilitation. She is determined to go back to work in her home office as soon as possible.

OT: "Hello, Sarah. I am covering for your regular OT to provide your afternoon therapy. I am here to practice with you how to put on socks and shoes."

SARAH: "Ohhhh. I am really tired—it's Friday at 4:00 p.m. My family is visiting this evening, and anyway, I can already put on my shoes and socks."

OT: "So, you are not sure if you want to participate in OT today." (Complex reflection)

TABLE 5.2

Examples of Integrating MI to Promote Self-Management

MI approaches	Examples
Open-ended questions	"Tell me what it means to attend this event."
	"What have you tried to feel comfortable meeting people you haven't seen since your MS diagnosis?"
	"How do you feel about meeting new people?"
Affirmation	"You are thoughtful about how fatigue affects your energy at different times during the day."
	"You are determined to go to the event, and you came up with a solid plan."
Reflections	"It is frustrating when people stare at you when you use your scooter."
	"It makes you anxious not knowing whether the venue is accessible or not."
Summarizing	"This is a new experience for you, and with everything going on, you don't feel like you are ready to go. You are especially worried about what people might think of your disability. You think it would be helpful to brainstorm some ideas on how to talk about your disability, so you have those in your back pocket. Did I get it all?"
Information exchange (ask-offer-ask)	"Would it be OK if we spent 5 minutes talking about incontinence?" (Patient said yes.) "What have you tried so far that worked when going on outings?" (Ask)
	(Patient states that they don't know what will work for them.)
	"Would you like to hear strategies that other people try to deal with incontinence when they are outside of their home?" (Ask)
	Provide information such as not drinking before going out or wearing Depends to feel safe. (Offer)
	"What do you think about these ideas?" (Ask)
Action-planning	"What is one small, concrete action that you want to do in the next week?"
Using rulers	"On a scale of 0 to 10, how important is it for you to attend the event?" "On a scale of 0 to 10, how confident are you that you can deal with the concerns you have?"

Note: MI = motivational interviewing; MS = multiple sclerosis.

SARAH: "I would really prefer not to have OT this afternoon."

OT: "I understand. Before I go, may I ask you a question?" (Asking permission)

SARAH: "Sure."

OT: "What kinds of things will you need to do independently when you go home next week?" (Open-ended question)

SARAH: "Right now, I have trouble moving my operated leg, and I need to be able to get in and out of bed myself. I can't stand for more than 5 minutes, and I need to be able to at least heat up food for myself. I'm afraid of falling, so I'm worried about going from my bedroom upstairs to my office on the first floor. I used to go up and down the stairs all day, and I need to be able to do that at least once in the morning and once in the evening."

OT: "So, you have several activities that you need to do to manage independently once home." (Simple reflection) "Tell me more about what is the most important for you to work on right now." (Open-ended question)

SARAH: "Well, getting in and out of bed. I live alone, so I need to be able to get in and out of bed safely by myself to go to the bathroom or the commode. If I can do it safely, it will save me from hiring someone to help me during the night."

OT: "So, you want to be able to confidently get in and out of bed during the night." (Complex reflection)

SARAH: "Yes, I am not sure that I can get in and out of bed at night, and that makes me anxious. I don't want to have to wear a diaper or worry that I might fall if I get up to go to the bathroom."

OT: "It would be a load off your mind if you could get in and out of bed yourself. If you can muster the energy, we can work on getting in and out of bed right now." (Complex reflection, asking permission)

SARAH: "OK, I would like to do that."

OT: "Talk me through what you can do, and show me where you get stuck and what you have tried."

[Practice . . .]

Sarah demonstrates her current abilities. She gets stuck with getting her operated leg in and out of the bed. The OT problem-solves options with the patient, and they test out using a towel to support her leg as she guides it gently in and out of the bed. Sarah is excited to do this on her own. The OT shares with permission that she could also use a leg lifter, which is easier than using a towel, and suggests that she try this with her regular OT on Monday. (Information exchange)

SARAH: "That was very helpful. I'm surprised I can get in and out myself now. It's a relief to me."

OT: "Today, you were persistent, and problem-solved actively to figure out a solution for getting in and out of bed yourself. Your progress surprised you. You still have challenges you would like to address to be independent at home. What is your next step before going home?" (Affirmation, complex reflection, summary, ending with an open-ended question)

SARAH: "I want to practice getting in and out of bed to make sure I can do it. Then I want to figure out a way to at least warm food at home."

OT: "Sounds like you have a clear plan. I encourage you to share these ideas with your OT so that you can work on them before you go home. Nice to work with you."

The OT did not push or demand that the patient participate when they entered the room for therapy. They listened to the patient, who wanted to rest up for visitors, and to her belief that the planned task was not needed or valuable. Rather than creating discord, the OT inquired about what was important to the patient to address before going home and guided her to identify one task that could be worked on in the moment. When it was a task of interest, the patient immediately engaged. During the practice session, the OT did not give tips and suggestions throughout. They allowed the patient to work on the task and then problem-solved with her when she was stuck and asked for permission before guiding her to try an assistive device that might help her get in and out of bed independently.

CASE 2

Ahn is a 68-year-old woman who had surgery for L2 compression fracture. Her precautions immediately post-surgery limit all bending and twisting. She was recently discharged with a lot of pain. She takes pride in helping care for her 8-year-old grandson. Her daughter is currently off work to assist her as she is recovering. Ahn was seen at home for home health OT.

OT: "Ahn, we had a very busy session today, and you fully participated in every activity. Can we talk about how the activities today worked for you?" (Affirmation, asking permission)

AHN: "Sure, I am happy to. . . . I realized from the practice with the long-handled equipment and going from sitting to standing how bad my pain is. The suggestions and tips helped, but I am going to need more practice. The breathing relaxation tape reduced my pain a little bit which was a relief, and I was pleasantly surprised that just thinking and breathing could leave me feeling less pain."

OT: "So, the breathing tape gave you hope of gaining control of your pain." (Complex reflection)

AHN: "Yes, I think the other activities were important, but I will get better quicker if I have less pain."

OT: "So how could the breathing exercises make your life easier right now?" (Open-ended question)

AHN: "If I could get pain relief even once a day, it would raise my spirits and I would feel less frustrated and worried about being a burden to my daughter and son-in-law."

OT: "Any break from the pain would be welcome." (Simple reflection)

AHN: "Yes, that is very true."

OT: "It is hard for you to complete daily activities because of the doctor's restrictions and because you are experiencing a great deal of pain. You have a strong desire to regain your independence as you do not want to be a burden to your daughter and son-in-law. You saw value in the activities today, yet the most important for your progress and morale is the breathing practice because it gives hope you can control your pain. Did I get it all?" (Summary)

AHN: "Yes, you did. I need to get control of my pain."

OT: "I encourage my patients to practice something between sessions. You mentioned that getting pain relief even once a day would help you manage, and I wonder how you could imagine doing this." (Action-planning, simple reflection, open-ended question)

AHN: "I think I would like to use the 6-minute relaxation script we practiced today."

OT: "So, many people find it helpful to make a specific plan, in your case to increase independence and pain control. Would that work for you?" (Asking permission)

AHN: "Yes, I would like to listen to the relaxation tape we tried earlier."

OT: "When will you listen?" (Action-planning)

AHN: "Right before I get out of bed."

OT: "How often will you listen to the tape?" (Action-planning)

AHN: "Once a day, so twice before you come again on Friday."

OT: "So, you will listen to the 6-minute relaxation tape before getting out of bed once a day, twice before our Friday session." (Simple reflection)

AHN: "Yes."

OT: "I will leave the CD for you to borrow. Good luck, and see you Friday."

The OT ended the session by getting the patient's perspective on what was helpful. She expected the patient to find the long-handled equipment most helpful as it would assist her in gaining independence. When given a choice, the patient reported she found the 6-minute relaxation tape most useful because it offered pain relief. To facilitate practice between sessions, the OT offered the patient an opportunity to set an action plan. In the next session, the OT learned that the patient met the action plan and found the tape helpful with pain management.

Conclusion

Both MI and self-management focus on the active role of patients in their care. Effective self-management is essential to optimizing health outcomes for people with chronic conditions. Self-management skills and tasks allow patients to build skills, knowledge, and confidence in managing their medical condition and lives. MI provides a set of skills and principles that can guide clinicians to work in a collaborative relationship with their patients and communicate to promote self-management. MI spirit lays the foundation for self-management and helps rehabilitation clinicians to share power, to accept patients where they are, to identify strengths, and to feel the urge to help. The four MI tasks guide clinicians in their work helping patients attain self-management skills. MI offers specific communication skills to engage patients in building self-management skills and help them rebuild their life after rehabilitation.

References

Afshin, A., Sur, P. J., Fay, K. A., Cornaby, L., Ferrara, G., Salama, J. S., Mullany, E. C., Abate, K. H., Abbafati, C., Abebe, Z., Afarideh, M., Aggarwal, A., Agrawal, S., Akinyemiju, T., Alahdab, F., Bacha, U., Bachman, V. F., Badali, H., Badawi, A., . . . Murray, C. J. L. (2019). Health effects of dietary risks in 195 countries, 1990–2017: A systematic analysis for the Global Burden of Disease Study 2017. *Lancet, 393*(10184), 1958–1972. https://doi.org/10.1016/S0140-6736(19)30041-8

Algurén, B., Fridlund, B., Cieza, A., Sunnerhagen, K. S., & Christensson, L. (2012). Factors associated with health-related quality of life after stroke: A 1-year prospective cohort study. *Neurorehabilitation and Neural Repair, 26*(3), 266–274.

Ang, S. (2019). How social participation benefits the chronically ill: Self-management as a mediating pathway. *Journal of Aging and Health, 31*(7), 1134–1154. https://doi.org/10.1177/08982 64318761909

Bamm, E. L., Rosenbaum, P., Wilkins, S., Stratford, P., & Mahlberg, N. (2015). Exploring client-centered care experiences in in-patient rehabilitation settings. *Global Qualitative Nursing Research, 2*, 2333393615582036. https://doi.org/10.1177/2333393615582036

Barlow, J., Wright, C., Sheasby, J., Turner, A., & Hainsworth, J. (2002). Self-management approaches for people with chronic conditions: A review. *Patient Education and Counseling, 48*(2), 177–187.

Battersby, M., Von Korff, M., Schaefer, J., Davis, C., Ludman, E., Greene, S. M., Parkerton, M., & Wagner, E. H. (2010). Twelve evidence-based principles for implementing self-management support in primary care. *Joint Commission Journal on Quality and Patient Safety, 36*(12), 561–570.

Billinger, S. A., Arena, R., Bernhardt, J., Eng, J. J., Franklin, B. A., Johnson, C. M., MacKay-Lyons, M., Macko, R. F., Mead, G. E., Roth, E. J., Shaughnessy, M., & Tang, A. (2014). Physical activity and exercise recommendations for stroke survivors: A statement for healthcare professionals from the American Heart Association/American Stroke Association. *Stroke, 45*(8), 2532–2553. https://doi.org/10.1161/STR.0000000000000022

Centers for Disease Control and Prevention. (2020, June 25). *Support and education for patient disease management.* Retrieved May 22, 2022, from https://www.cdc.gov/dhdsp/pubs/guides/best-practices/self-management.htm

Clifford, D., & Curtis, L. (2015). *Motivational interviewing in nutrition and fitness.* Guilford Press.

Ezekiel, L., Collett, J., Mayo, N. E., Pang, L., Field, L., & Dawes, H. (2019). Factors associated with participation in life situations for adults with stroke: A systematic review. *Archives of Physical Medicine and Rehabilitation, 100*(5), 945–955. https://doi.org/10.1016/j.apmr.2018.06.017

Feng, Z., Cramm, J. M., & Nieboer, A. P. (2020). Social participation is an important health behaviour for health and quality of life among chronically ill older Chinese people. *BMC Geriatrics, 20*(1), Article 299. https://doi.org/10.1186/s12877-020-01713-6

Ginis, K. A. M., van der Ploeg, H. P., Foster, C., Lai, B., McBride, C. B., Ng, K., Pratt, M., Shirazipour, C. H., Smith, B., Vásquez, P. M., & Heath, G. W. (2021). Participation of people living with disabilities in physical activity: A global perspective. *Lancet, 398*(10298), 443–455. https://doi.org/10.1016/S0140-6736(21)01164-8

Guilcher, S. J. T., Everall, A. C., Patel, T., Packer, T. L., Hitzig, S. L., & Lofters, A. K. (2019). Medication adherence for persons with spinal cord injury and dysfunction from the perspectives of healthcare providers: A qualitative study. *The Journal of Spinal Cord Medicine, 42*(S1), 215–225. https://doi.org/10.1080/10790268.2019.1637644

Jones, F., Riazi, A., & Norris, M. (2013). Self-management after stroke: Time for some more questions? *Disability and Rehabilitation, 35*(3), 257–264. https://doi.org/10.3109/09638288.2012.691938

Loft, M. I., Martinsen, B., Esbensen, B. A., Mathiesen, L. L., Iversen, H. K., & Poulsen, I. (2019). Call for human contact and support: An interview study exploring patients' experiences with inpatient stroke rehabilitation and their perception of nurses' and nurse assistants' roles and functions. *Disability and Rehabilitation, 41*(4), 396–404. https://doi.org/10.1080/09638288.2017.1393698

Miller, W. R., & Moyers, T. B. (2021). *Effective psychotherapists: Clinical skills that improve client outcomes* (1st ed.). Guilford Press.

Miller, W. R., & Rollnick, S. (2013). *Motivational interviewing: Helping people change* (3rd ed.). Guilford Press.

Miller, W. R., & Rollnick, S. (2023). *Motivational interviewing: Helping people change and grow* (4th ed.). Guilford Publications.

Palstam, A., Sjödin, A., & Sunnerhagen, K. S. (2019). Participation and autonomy five years after stroke: A longitudinal observational study. *PLOS ONE, 14*(7), Article e0219513. https://doi.org/10.1371/journal.pone.0219513

Peoples, H., Satink, T., & Steultjens, E. (2011). Stroke survivors' experiences of rehabilitation: A systematic review of qualitative studies. *Scandinavian Journal of Occupational Therapy, 18*(3), 163–171. https://doi.org/10.3109/11038128.2010.509887

Rimmer, J. H., Riley, B., Wang, E., Rauworth, A., & Jurkowski, J. (2004). Physical activity participation among persons with disabilities: Barriers and facilitators. *American Journal of Preventive Medicine, 26*(5), 419–425. https://doi.org/10.1016/j.amepre.2004.02.002

Ruppar, T. M., Cooper, P. S., Mehr, D. R., Delgado, J. M., & Dunbar-Jacob, J. M. (2016). Medication adherence interventions improve heart failure mortality and readmission rates: Systematic review and meta-analysis of controlled trials. *Journal of the American Heart Association, 5*(6), Article e002606. https://doi.org/10.1161/JAHA.115.002606

Scelza, W. M., Kalpakjian, C. Z., Zemper, E. D., & Tate, D. G. (2005). Perceived barriers to exercise in people with spinal cord injury. *American Journal of Physical Medicine & Rehabilitation, 84*(8), 576–583. https://doi.org/10.1097/01.phm.0000171172.96290.67

6   Rehabilitation Team Dynamics
Emily Markley and Ruth Grenoble

What Is the Rehabilitation Team?

Team-based medical care began after World War II in response to an increased complexity of medical conditions and recovery courses due to soldiers surviving injuries from which they likely would have previously died (Baldwin, 1996; Strasser et al., 2008). Approaches to healthcare, and particularly in rehabilitation medicine, have progressed over the years from a single-discipline model in which the physician was the primary deliverer of care to at least a multidisciplinary model. Multidisciplinary models mean that more than one discipline is involved in the healthcare, with each discipline remaining essentially siloed. Many rehabilitation clinics or facilities now provide interdisciplinary care, which describes more than one discipline collaborating to solve a problem as it arises. Team approaches are successful in part due to the ability of rehabilitation teams to reduce the separation between healthcare and daily life (Karol, 2014).

The current movement in rehabilitation is toward transdisciplinary care, which describes that multiple disciplines collaborate throughout the rehabilitation process, bringing their unique knowledge and expertise to create a holistic approach to patient care. In this model, there are often inherent overlaps between care provided by different disciplines, and therefore an ongoing need for providers in various

Emily Markley and Ruth Grenoble, *Rehabilitation Team Dynamics* In: *Motivational Interviewing in Medical Rehabilitation.*
Edited by: Nicole Schechter, Connie Jacocks, Lester Butt, and Stephen T. Wegener, Oxford University Press.
© Oxford University Press 2024. DOI: 10.1093/oso/9780197748268.003.0007

disciplines to collaborate regarding the patient/care recipient (Karol, 2014; Malec, 2013). Importantly, a transdisciplinary approach also identifies that patients be considered as core members of their care teams and that teams consider patient progress based on the functional area/category rather than by discipline (Karol, 2014).

Both interdisciplinary and transdisciplinary teams are well suited to integrate motivational interviewing (MI) as a best practice for successful rehabilitative care. Specifically, MI allows for extremely patient-centric care, with the patient as an active participant in goal-setting rather than a passive recipient of rehabilitation interventions. The MI spirit and skills are also very useful in guiding interactions between team members. This is especially important on interdisciplinary and transdisciplinary teams, where overlapping competencies and roles can pose challenges.

The composition of rehabilitation teams varies across settings and systems of care and tends to include the following disciplines (Behm & Gray, 2012; Karol, 2014; Strasser et al., 2008):

- Physicians (MD, DO), nurse practitioners, and physician assistants, all typically specialized in rehabilitation-related areas such as physical medicine and rehabilitation, neurology, or geriatrics, though other specialty providers may also participate.
- Rehabilitation therapy services such as physical therapists (PTs) and PT assistants, occupational therapists (OTs) and OT assistants, and speech and language pathologists.
- Direct care/front-line nursing staff such as registered nurses (RNs), certified nursing assistants (CNAs), and/or licensed practical nurses, depending on setting and state licensure requirements.
- Other allied health professionals such as certified therapeutic recreation specialists, registered dieticians, pharmacists, respiratory therapists, peer counselors, and chaplains.
- Mental health professionals such as rehabilitation psychologists and/or neuropsychologists.
- Case management/care coordination/discharge planning staff such as social workers and/or RN case managers.
- Note that other medical and mental health specialists such as pulmonologists, infectious disease specialists, gastroenterologists, otolaryngologists, neuropsychiatrists, neuro-optometrists, vocational rehabilitation professionals, and other relevant specialists may be included in patient care delivery depending on setting; and participation in interdisciplinary team discussions will vary based on setting.

Roles and responsibilities of various team members are often setting-specific based on the cultural norms of the particular system of care. In general, traditional team models formally place the physician in the position of team "leader," and the physician leader often has explicit organizational leadership responsibilities. However, other team members can have significant implicit leadership roles and responsibilities, based on specific patient needs or the team member's ability to appreciate group process. Successful teams can function without hierarchical structures, as long as roles and responsibilities are delineated and understood/agreed upon by the team as a whole.

What Are the Common Rehabilitation Team Challenges, and Why Do These Matter?

When functioning at their prime, rehabilitation teams can provide a supportive and patient-centric interpersonal environment in which a patient can achieve optimal recovery outcomes and all disciplines are able to contribute and communicate effectively. Although rehabilitation teams often function successfully, challenges of team-based care do exist. Just like clinician use of MI with patients enhances patient outcomes and patient experience/satisfaction, team members' use of MI with one another can be helpful in navigating the difficulties that teams encounter. These skills can help teams overcome challenges related to communication styles, values, and role responsibilities.

In general, rehabilitation professionals are often drawn to the field because they are eager to support those with disabilities. If one spends time in any rehabilitation setting, one will realize that team members tend to be naturally filled with compassion. Even with this foundation, challenges in team interpersonal dynamics, including differences in communication styles (Nancarrow et al., 2013) and value systems, do exist. When not successfully navigated, these issues can negatively impact patient care and team morale.

COMMUNICATION STYLE DIFFERENCES

Depending on cultural factors, family systems, geographical factors, and other domains of a person's background, individual team members are comfortable with varying levels of directness (Mole et al., 2016). Some team members may perceive direct feedback as personal criticism, while the deliverer believes they are communicating directly and assertively. Such differences, if not openly discussed or if disrespected, can cause discord among team members and lead to diminished communication overall. MI can be used to elicit information from colleagues around preferred styles of communication. MI can also be used to work with a particular colleague on using a different type of communication that works better for the rest of the team.

As described in Chapter 1, some individuals use a directing style of communication, some use a following style of communication, and others use a guiding style of communication. MI encourages the use of a refined guiding style when we seek collaboration—be that with patients or colleagues. If rehabilitation professionals are aiming for a guiding style in their work with patients, it builds this skill by using the guiding style when interacting with their peers. Further, modeling a guiding style encourages peers with more directive styles to adapt and change to a style that is more effective in collaborative teams. Use of open-ended questions and reflecting feeling when tensions arise from different styles can move the team in a positive direction.

VALUE SYSTEM DIFFERENCES

Team members may also have different value systems than their colleagues and their patients, which can lead to conflict. For example, one team member may value individualism very highly, while another team member may value collectivism. This may lead to challenges between the team members when structuring a treatment plan for a patient who appears to be less motivated toward functional independence and more interested in relying on their grown children for assistance. Another example is when two team members value marriage differently and struggle to communicate with one another about a patient who opts to receive care from an ex-spouse. Importantly, no value system is "right" or "wrong." Similar to how teams need to understand patients' value systems to provide optimal care, team members must seek to understand their own values and their colleagues' values to collaborate as a unit.

PATIENT MISCONCEPTIONS AROUND TEAM LEADERSHIP STRUCTURE

Misconceptions around leadership structures or hierarchies within the team can also affect the quality of care delivered to patients and team morale. Such confusion can occur for patients and for team members themselves. Traditionally, the physician is considered the leader of the team, and so patients may highly value a physician's recommendations. At times patients may weigh physicians' opinions over those of other team members. For other myriad reasons, a patient may weigh another team member's perspective more highly than that of others, thereby creating the same type of team dynamic. Therefore, it is essential that teams discuss and come to a consensus on treatment goals, approaches, and discharge plans before communicating with the patient.

TEAM MISCONCEPTIONS AROUND OVERLAPPING COMPETENCIES

Particularly in transdisciplinary teams there are opportunities for overlapping competencies and expertise, which can create confusion around who is responsible for addressing specific patient symptoms or problems. For example, several disciplines have expertise in assessing cognitive impairment. This is not inherently conflictual, and in fact multiple sets of observations and conclusions from different disciplines can serve the patient well. As an example, a patient may score differently on similar cognitive measures administered by two separate clinicians (e.g., speech language pathology, neuropsychology). By discussing the patient's approach, possible mitigating factors, and clinical observations, score discrepancies can be explored and provide better understanding of the patient's abilities and performance variables. This in turn can become an advantage for treatment planning. It is imperative that team members are able to collectively plan for assessment and then after the fact discuss assessment approaches, patient observations, and results so that no team member perceives that another is infringing on a specific domain.

TEAM MISALIGNMENT AROUND RESPONSIBILITIES

Another common challenge for teams is when members do not align in perspectives on which team member or discipline is responsible for which patient care tasks. Often, such misalignment occurs because of lack of communication or miscommunications. Other times, such misalignment occurs because team members have low efficacy in their own ability to complete certain duties or low efficacy in others' abilities to complete certain duties. For example, PTs may expect that patients are dressed, out of bed, and ready for therapy by their scheduled session. Nurses may be able to do this easily for some patients. However, for patients who require significant physical assistance for a variety of reasons, the nurse may hesitate to transfer the patient due to lack of confidence in their own abilities. Overt communication between nurses and PTs regarding expectations for each patient, self-efficacy for tasks related to each patient, and opportunities for education between disciplines will improve this challenge.

READER REFLECTION QUESTIONS

The aforementioned challenges are not comprehensive. Take a moment and consider your own experiences of team-based challenges by reading and responding to all or some of the following questions:

- What are the primary challenges you've faced at the team level?
- How were these issues managed? How were these issues not managed well?
- What role did you play in their resolution or implicit continuation?
- What can you envision yourself doing when these issues next emerge?
- How can you positively impact the team culture?
- How can you invite others to so participate?

How Is MI Helpful for Navigating Rehabilitation Team Challenges?

MI spirit and skills can be used when teams encounter the above challenges. Use of MI can also help an interdisciplinary or transdisciplinary team foster a culture of mutual respect, collaboration, and willingness to give and receive constructive feedback. The spirit and skills of MI facilitate communication and help with behavior change that may be necessary by team members. This section will highlight aspects of the MI spirit and MI skills that may be particularly useful to the rehabilitation team. We will provide specific examples from Video 7, "MI and the Rehab Team," which can be found on the Rehabilitation Engagement Collaborative (REC) website (https://www.rehabengage.org/). We encourage all readers to watch this video, which shows a team using the MI spirit and skills during a team conference and how it can facilitate a respectful and effective discussion in a challenging situation.

The MI spirit outlined by the principles of partnership, acceptance, compassion, and empowerment forms the foundation of the method and is crucial in the context of managing team dynamics. Please review Chapter 1 for a complete overview of the MI spirit. Partnership is applied when team members view one another as not only complementary but essential in providing optimal patient care. An example of partnership in the team context is a PT acknowledging the important work that a nurse has done to get the patient out of bed and ready for therapies by 8:00 a.m. Demonstrating acceptance in the team context may involve being nonjudgmental of colleagues who have different backgrounds or perspectives from you.

Compassion may be especially important during difficult discussions with a team member who is overwhelmed. Leading with compassion can support a productive conversation even if it contains constructive feedback. The principle of *empowerment* described in Miller & Rollnick's (2023) newest publication as calling forth others' strengths and perspectives, is especially important when discussing differing opinions on treatment or discharge plans. For example, seeking to understand colleagues' perspectives prior to giving your own perspective can be helpful if the goal is collaborative, interdisciplinary/transdisciplinary care. Though it is most beneficial when all team members approach interdisciplinary or transdisciplinary work with the MI spirit, this is not always realistic. That said, one person's conscious decision to infuse the MI spirit in a difficult conversation can prompt an entire team to change course.

The MI skills of open-ended questions, affirmations, reflections, and summaries are also very useful in team communications. Open-ended questions can be used to demonstrate one's openness and interest in hearing the input of each team member, allowing each team member to feel heard and valued. In the aforementioned REC video, we observe a team member using a closed-ended question ("I'm sure you've all seen [the patient's behavior] too, right?") to elicit input from the broader team. An open-ended question like "Therapists, what are you noticing?" will help team members feel valued because it invites a greater opportunity to provide individual perspectives and greater detail. Another example is when a physician asks the team "What are some of the things we need to do to get him ready for discharge?" This conveys the physician's valuing of the other team members and helps to move the team forward to an action plan.

Using affirmations with a colleague serves as a signal that you are aware of, and believe in, their strengths. As seen in the REC video, the physician is able to couch concerns about the team's hesitancy to discharge the patient in the context of an affirmation, that, above all, the team cares about the patient: "You're all obviously very concerned about Johnny and his family, and you care about what happens to him after discharge." This summary helped to shore up the team's confidence and remind the team of its unified core values. Generally, people have an easier time hearing a differing opinion after their character has been validated.

In one portion of the video, a PT notices that the conversation has become unhelpful because the team is stuck harping on concerns about discharging the patient to another facility. She uses a reflection to acknowledge her colleagues' perspectives, which helps them to feel heard, and then uses an open-ended question to shift the conversation productively, "I wonder if we can identify some optimal options for this patient?" Another example is when a team member reflects the team's frustrations with the patient's barriers to engagement and reflects how the patient must be feeling. This validates the team's frustration and simultaneously creates compassion for the patient.

Summaries gather together each team member's input and create momentum for the team's next steps or action plan. In the REC video, the psychologist synthesizes the team's concerns about this particular patient's discharge plan and reminds the team that there is a unified goal in helping the patient. She says, "This is a challenging case, and at the same time it is clear that we all want what's best for him. There are three things that I've heard everyone talking about." Summaries are improved when they end in open-ended questions, which invite additional input and other perspectives. A question like "What should we talk about first?" allows other team members to guide the conversation, emphasizing that others' perspectives are valued. Summaries like this one lead to team members feeling heard, the team feeling cohesive, and improved chances for team follow-through.

READER REFLECTION QUESTIONS

Before you go on, stop and consider:

- Which aspects of MI spirit or which MI skills are feasible for you to use when working with your team members?
- In what team contexts would you like to incorporate MI? Team meetings? One-on-one team communications?
- What would you like to commit to in terms of increasing your strategic use of a certain MI skill or two in the context of team dynamics?

Case Examples

Below are two case examples which highlight the use of specific MI skills within a rehabilitation interdisciplinary team environment.

CASE I

The first example involves the team treating a White male ("Jim") in his early 20s who suffered a severe traumatic brain injury and orthopedic injuries as a result of a helmeted motorcycle accident. Jim is receiving acute inpatient rehabilitation. This conversation occurred during interdisciplinary team rounds, which the patient did not attend.

> PHYSICIAN: "I look forward to hearing everyone's perspective on this patient and working together to address any challenges. Where should we begin?" (Open-ended question)

NURSE: "Well, we have really had a tough time with Jim this week."

OT: "Agreed, we have had trouble getting him to participate too since he is so behavioral."

PSYCHOLOGIST: "I'd love to take a step back and help figure out how we can get through some of Jim's barriers. What types of situations have been challenging this week?" (Open-ended question)

NURSE: "Our staff is just getting so burnt out with him. He's really inappropriate and mean, and we just don't feel safe."

PT: "In PT sessions this week he has made me really uncomfortable as well."

OT: "Agreed. I can hardly get anything accomplished in my sessions since I am just redirecting him for the first half or more of our sessions."

SOCIAL WORKER: "It sounds like Jim is requiring a lot of effort and energy in the nursing care settings and during therapy sessions. Is that a fair statement?" (Summary)

ALL: "Yes, that sounds right."

PHYSICIAN: Tell me about a time over the last few days when the interaction with Jim was challenging and you were able to find a solution. (Open-ended question)

PT: "Actually, I would be happy to share something from today. I was trying to work with Jim on transfers today, and he was swearing a lot and just getting really upset when I tried to get through our session."

PSYCHOLOGIST: "He was having really strong reactions to the interventions you were trying." (Reflection)

PT: "Yes, and since it kept getting worse, I just backed off for a while and let him cool off."

OT: "You thought of a solution in the moment. You're creative and adaptable." (Affirmation)

PT: "Thanks! Yes, I didn't want to waste an entire session getting into a power struggle with him."

NURSE: "What seemed to lead up to the times when Jim was swearing? That's been happening with me too." (Open-ended question)

PT: "I think when I touched his trunk or legs to try to reposition him, that seemed to not go very well."

NURSE: "The physical touch was upsetting to him." (Reflection)

PT: "Yes, so I tried to give him lots of warning and cueing when I would be needing to touch him, which seemed to help."

NURSE: "Maybe it would be helpful to track Jim's triggers and solutions that we find to share as a team."

OT: "That's a great idea. What can we do to keep track of this?" (Open-ended question)

PSYCHOLOGY: "This team is really committed to working together to find a way to best meet Jim's needs." (Affirmation). "Just to confirm, I am hearing that Jim is responding to physical touch pretty strongly and that giving him cues and using verbal descriptions of the touch we are planning has been helpful in reducing his swearing during sessions." (Summary)

PT: "Yes, that seems accurate."

SOCIAL WORKER: "Well this is great information. I'd like to propose that we start to have our CNA staff track what leads up to negative verbal reactions. How does that sound?" (Summary)

ALL: "Great! Seems like that will give us some good information to help Jim."

PHYSICIAN: "Wonderful. We will provide some specific tools to our CNA staff for tracking. And I want to acknowledge PT's quick thinking when it came to behavior management today. The team is being really creative and thoughtful about this case. Thanks, everyone." (Affirmation)

Case 1 Debrief

In this example, note that the psychologist does not criticize the OT for using the term *behavioral* but rather uses a summary to validate the team's concerns and an open-ended question to guide the conversation in a new direction. The OT, social worker, and physician also offer affirmations of the work being done by other team members. Notice that at various points different team members take the lead of the conversation and that all are able to utilize MI skills. When the team is grounded in the MI spirit and demonstrates compassion for one another and acceptance of the members' perspectives, the discussion is fruitful, which ultimately leads to optimized patient-centered care.

CASE 2

The next example involves a conversation between two team members outside of rounds.

PT: "Hi Dr. Star, do you have a minute to chat?"

PHYSICIAN: "Yes, of course! Please come in."

PT: "Thank you. I'd love to share some feedback about rounds this week."

PHYSICIAN: "Great—appreciate your input."

PT: "Well, it was a difficult meeting, and I am trying to figure out what exactly was tough for me."

PHYSICIAN: "Something about rounds this week did not go the way you had hoped." (Reflection)

PT: "Yes, it was challenging for me because I felt like my feedback was not being considered."

PHYSICIAN: "You didn't feel heard." (Reflection)

PT: "Right. Tell me a little bit about your overall style when it comes to team rounds and information sharing?" (Open-ended question)

PHYSICIAN: "That's a great question, and I don't know that I have thought about that. I think my style is to hear from other members of the team, and I also know that I can sometimes rush through things because I want to allot adequate time to discuss all the patients on our list."

PT: "You want and value input from each team member, and sometimes time constraints can be a challenge given that we have quite a few patients to discuss." (Reflection)

PHYSICIAN: "Exactly. Can you help me understand more about your experience in rounds this week?" (Open-ended question)

PT: "There were certainly moments when I felt like there was more I wanted to say. And I was hoping to get feedback from the team on how to best work with the patient in Room 14. I am also not a very outgoing person, so it can be difficult for me to speak in a group setting like team rounds."

PHYSICIAN: "Here is what I have heard so far. Tell me if I've missed something. You have valuable feedback you'd like to offer at rounds and perspectives of other team members you'd like to hear to help guide your work with patients. You also shared that you are not always comfortable speaking up in groups." (Summary)

PT: "That sums it up pretty well."

PHYSICIAN: "What can we do to move forward and feel more like we are collaborating in team rounds?" (Open-ended question)

PT: "If we can have some time before moving from one patient to the next and allow more time for others to share their thoughts, that would be great."

PHYSICIAN: "Great ideas—you are committed to making our team meetings more effective." (Affirmation) "As you said, let me know if there is a patient who might need more in-depth discussion." (Reflection)

PT: "Thank you! I appreciate your willingness to have difficult discussions to improve our team." (Affirmation)

Case 2 Debrief

In this example, both parties use MI skills throughout the discussion in an attempt to understand one another and the "stuck points" that are getting in the way of effective team communication. The spirit of empowerment is seen when both the PT and physician seek to understand the other's perspective as a means to support and encourage. The physician uses an open-ended question to elicit more information around the PT's experience and many reflections and summaries to help the PT feel heard in this meeting, especially because the PT did not feel heard during rounds. The PT uses a powerful affirmation at the end of the conversation, which will likely increase the physician's desire to be open in the future.

READER REFLECTION QUESTION

• How do you think MI might be useful to you and your team?

Summary

Working within an interdisciplinary or transdisciplinary team allows for patients to receive comprehensive expert care across multiple disciplines in what often is their greatest time of need. There are, however, a variety of challenges faced by the treatment teams. The same MI spirit and skills that are useful to engage our patients are also useful when working with our colleagues in one-on-one relationships and in team meetings. When individual team members use MI, the team will be more capable of joining together to deliver the highest-quality patient-centered care.

References

Baldwin, D. C., Jr. (1996). Some historical notes on interdisciplinary and interprofessional education and practice in healthcare in the USA. *Journal of Interprofessional Care, 10*(2), 173–187.

Behm, J., & Gray, N. (2012). *Rehabilitation nursing: A contemporary approach to practice.* Jones & Bartlett Learning.

Karol, R. L. (2014). Team models in neurorehabilitation: Structure, function, and culture change. *NeuroRehabilitation, 34*, 655–669. https://doi.org/10.3233/NRE-141080

Malec, J. F. (2013). Posthospital rehabilitation. In N. D. Zasler, D. I. Katz, & R. D. Zafonte (Eds.), *Brain injury medicine* (pp. 1288–1301). Demos Medical Publishing.

Miller, W. R. & Rollnick, S. (2023). *Motivational interviewing: Helping people change and grow.* Guilford Publications.

Mole, T. B., Begum, H., Cooper-Moss, N., Wheelhouse, R., MacKeith, P., Sanders, T., & Wass, V. (2016). Limits of "patient-centredness": Valuing contextually specific communication patterns. *Medical Education, 50*(3), 359–369. https://doi.org/10.1111/medu.12946

Nancarrow, S. A., Booth, A., Ariss, S., Smith, T., Enderby, P., & Roots, A. (2013). Ten principles of good interdisciplinary team work. *Human Resources for Health*, *11*, Article 19. https://doi.org/10.1186/1478-4491-11-19

Strasser, D. C., Uomoto, J. M., & Smits, S. J. (2008). The interdisciplinary team and polytrauma rehabilitation: Prescription for partnership. *Archives of Physical Medicine and Rehabilitation*, *89*(1), 179–181. https://doi.org/10.1016/j.apmr.2007.06.774

7 Transitions Between Treatment Settings

Sarah Horan and Allie Hamilton

Introduction

One of life's certainties is change. This is undoubtedly true for all rehabilitation patients and their families as they move from one care setting to their next life phase. In this chapter, the authors' intentions are multifactorial. One goal is to more fully describe common patient factors involved in these inevitable changes, illustrating issues that typically emerge when patients contemplate changing milieus. Consequently, topics such as momentum, resources, relationships, patient understanding, and coordination between facilities are broached.

An additional aim is to examine how motivational interviewing (MI) values, spirit, and skills can better support our patients through changes that occur during transitions of care. The MI spirit involves embracing patient autonomy, coupled with compassion, empowerment, and creation of a collaborative partnership. MI skills that facilitate constructive movement are illustrated via the use of OARS (open-ended questions, affirmations, reflections. and summaries).

Through the use of several clinical case examples, the authors examine how these MI features can facilitate constructive movement, promote patient understanding, and establish the aforementioned collaborative partnership. For a more detailed discussion of MI spirit, values, and skills, please refer to Miller and Rollnick's work

Sarah Horan and Allie Hamilton, *Transitions Between Treatment Settings* In: *Motivational Interviewing in Medical Rehabilitation*. Edited by: Nicole Schechter, Connie Jacocks, Lester Butt, and Stephen T. Wegener, Oxford University Press. © Oxford University Press 2024. DOI: 10.1093/oso/9780197748268.003.0008

(2013; 2023), the introductory chapters of this book, and https://www.rehabengage.org/, the latter using simulated video vignettes to demonstrate MI spirit and skills in action.

To ensure that readers understand the authors' meaning of care transitions, the following examples are offered: a patient's transition from home healthcare setting to long-term care facility, independent living to home healthcare, inpatient to outpatient, acute care to skilled nursing facility, outpatient to discharge, etc. While this list is representative of potential setting changes, it is assuredly not exhaustive in scope.

What Are Transitions Within Treatment Settings?

The professional literature illustrates how rehabilitative transitions for persons with complex needs leave them particularly vulnerable to clinical gaps and poor care quality (Coleman, 2003). Transitions from hospital to primary care for older patients with chronic disease lead to increased mortality and service use (Le Berre et al., 2017). Similar vulnerabilities are noted in individuals with neurologic conditions when transitioning care settings (Josephson, 2016). This research points to a need for healthcare providers to take specific interest in smoothing care transitions and helping patients to experience continuous high-level care throughout these changes.

The challenges presented to patients in transition of care provide the clinician with the opportunity to guide the patient toward a hopeful state of readiness and appreciation of the upcoming change. A collaborative relationship allows the clinician to appreciate the patient's inherent concerns, fears, and aspirations associated with this upcoming adjustment. The foundation of MI puts the patient in the center of the decision with the transition of care. The clinician examines the patient's ambivalence, strengths, priorities, and readiness for the change as they discuss the upcoming alteration in services. Specifically, MI skills of OARS and the spirit of MI are both relevant to help guide your patient through a transition of care and the rehabilitation challenges that accompany it.

How can we skillfully reach out to our patients and families to support them in partnership when faced with the aforementioned changes? Embracing the MI spirit means guiding conversations in a way that considers the patient's willingness for change, appreciates that the conversation is a true partnership, and understands that the clinician themselves can assist in evoking patient change. The rehabilitation clinician attempts to refrain from the *fixing reflex*, the tendency to use an authoritative stance where the patient is basically told what they should do and how to feel, as well as utilizing clinical expertise and training as evidence of this typically unproductive stance. The fixing reflex is, as a result, contrary to the true spirit of MI in that the patient's voice is overridden and/or not heard. The clinician is responsible not for demanding change but for guiding a patient to it, leaving them with their autonomy and sense of agency.

What Are the Challenges in Transitions of Treatment Settings?

The clinician seeks to understand the various aspects of the patient's life that contribute to the challenge with the transition and is accurately empathetic with these factors. Below are some supplemental patient factors at play when considering changing milieus.

MOMENTUM

Adjustment to a different schedule, a different set of goals generated by new clinicians, and a different set of processes within the new setting may leave clients feeling as if they have lost momentum, have slowed progress toward their goals, or have become confused about their rehabilitative trajectory.

In their pre-transition setting, patients have an established workflow that will now be interrupted by the change within their new environment and associated routine(s). The care provider has the opportunity to assist the patient in building their confidence, as well as envisioning this transition as a positive move. In an inpatient setting this may look like having conversations with the patient about the goals that they have set personally and how they have actively participated in achieving those goals. Utilizing MI spirit and skills, the rehabilitation professional can gently broach how the next treatment facility will help the patient build upon the goals that have yet to be achieved. Extra attention can be taken with having conversations about next steps, involving the patient in discussions early on about their care after discharge. Additionally, discussions with the patient to empower them in their own care can help to maintain a sense of momentum during transition.

PATIENT–HEALTHCARE PROVIDER RELATIONSHIPS

The client may have been invested with the current clinician and feel abandoned and anxious at the thought of establishing a new relationship(s). Conversely, the patient may have had a suboptimal relationship with the previous clinician that could affect their acceptance of the new treatment team. In the acute care setting, clinicians must consider the nature of their relationship with the patient and its potential impact on their patient's next setting. Lengths of stay are often short, leaving little time to build solid therapeutic collaborations, thereby placing a premium on utilizing the aforementioned MI spirit and skills to quickly create a collaborative, constructive, and egalitarian relationship. Conversely, in the long-term care setting a patient may grow a deep and lasting relationship with clinicians due to the consistency of their work together.

There are positives and negatives associated with each of these settings when it comes to transitioning care. Acute care lends its hand to a relatively quick transition, and this may be the patient's understanding, possibly making the transition easier. However, there is also risk that decisions appear hasty, with patients struggling to grasp the fast-paced transition of care and not building trusting relationships with the clinicians in charge of making these decisions. Again, stating this point, as a clinician in this setting, it is essential to make the patient the center of the decision-making process despite the ever-changing environment and professional demands.

Additionally, in the long-term setting, there is opportunity for a clinician to implement MI techniques through a long relationship with a patient, setting up the conversation for transition of care and evoking change far more naturally. Again, opportunity lies in long-term care for professionals to develop strong MI skills, as in all rehabilitative settings, to make these conversations easier, while minimizing a patient's tendency to rely only on the expertise of the clinician void of their voice and sense of involvement in the decision process.

RESOURCES

Patients may experience difficulties accessing resources required for the transition in care. Resources such as funds for hired personal care, accessible transportation, and capacity to organize and maintain a schedule when facilities utilize different technological services can prove monumental. These are just some aspects of transition that may be challenging. Again, in the acute care setting, facility resources may be limited for helping a patient navigate the community setting, thereby making this transition especially difficult. Patients may struggle to access transportation when their living situation has changed. A scarcity of financial resources can reflect another barrier to a patient's readiness to embrace change. They may not have finances to pay for private transportation, purchase specialty equipment, modify current living spaces, or hire personal care attendants. Rehabilitation professionals must recognize the unique way resources evidence either barriers or opportunities for a patient's transition of care. Again, through utilization of the MI spirit and skills, the clinician can far better appreciate their patient's concerns and unique perspectives and hopefully be a resource in the resolution of these issues.

PATIENT UNDERSTANDING

It is imperative for us, as rehabilitation professionals, to understand the world through our patients' eyes. As a result, how they understand the foundational underpinnings for the setting change is key. Through MI inquiry and listening, we obtain a glimpse into a deeper appreciation of the connotative meaning of the milieu change. Additionally, at times treatment teams can inaccurately assume that patients and families understand the details and specifics of medical care. For example, families may not understand what a functional goal is as opposed to a generalized strengthening goal. As a result, therapists need to fully explain that a patient's stay is predicated upon safety-related functional goals. In contrast, clinicians cannot justify keeping a patient on the inpatient side solely for strengthening. In an outpatient setting, insurance coverage could influence a provider's plan of care from high frequency to lower frequency and longer duration.

The explanation of these decisions regarding care programs and transitions will only strengthen the partnership between provider and patient. If the patient and family lack a big picture understanding of long-term goals and expectations, they may have a more difficult time adjusting when care settings change. Asking permission to share information such as this with a patient can help to harness the power of MI while still educating the patient and guiding them forward in the transition.

ROLE CONFLICTS

As rehabilitation clinicians, we need to think about our patients in a holistic way. Consequently, we must understand the competing obligations and roles our patients are experiencing. For example, how does their role and identification as parent change when their adult children become primary caregivers? Have they previously been the primary household income provider? Are they reluctant to transition home due to fears of their changing roles within their marriage?

A lack of resources, such as limitations in insurance coverage, paid time off from an employer, transportation, or even child care, are all factors that the patient may not have to coordinate or attend to as an inpatient but then become center stage at home. A patient's transition from inpatient to outpatient broadens their personal responsibility. Imagine the role change that occurs when a wife also becomes a primary caregiver, or a CEO in charge of a major business is now confronted with coordination, hiring, and managing personal caregivers. In these major life transitions, it is apparent that what may at first seem like resistance and denial is actually rooted in some very understandable life concerns. Using MI to inquire about how these factors play into our patients' acceptance of transition in care can assist in creating a smoother overall care transition.

COORDINATION OF CARE BETWEEN SETTINGS

It could well prove important to become the liaison between settings in deference to heightening the patient's understanding of their new setting, provide requisite information about this site, and even introduce new clinicians/caregivers if possible. This could prove most helpful in reducing anticipatory apprehensions, provide a link from present to the future, and thereby render the patient more comfortable with their new placement. Even if the patient is transitioning home, information related to home modifications, introduction to potential caregivers, etc., could be highly beneficial.

How Can MI Support Transitions of Treatment Settings?

We have an opportunity to facilitate conversations that are more collaborative during all of our interactions with our patients, knowing that eventually they will move on and out of our care. Utilizing MI skills, these conversations can be structured through active listening, asking open-ended questions, utilizing reflective listening, summarization, and informing the patient as small adjustments to their program are made. By having these conversations, the relationship is viewed as a partnership, trust is enhanced, and the patient is less likely to feel blindsided when a transition occurs.

The below case examples will first illustrate how a closed, disjointed exchange can happen between a clinician and their patient without use of MI skills. These conversations could be described as rushed or one-sided and unfortunately are far too common in some healthcare settings. Then, in contrast, MI spirit and skills are utilized to illustrate how this conversation could be better constructed with far improved patient–provider understanding and conjoint problem-solving.

Case Studies

CASE 1

The first example involves Jason, a patient who is discharging from inpatient rehabilitation to outpatient services. Jason was 22 years old when he sustained a spinal cord injury after diving from a boat into shallow water over the Fourth of July weekend.

Prior to his injury Jason played soccer in a recreational league, attended community college in hopes to become a math teacher, and played the drums in a band with friends from high school. He was renting a shared apartment and working part-time at a music store at the time of his injury.

The nature of his spinal cord injury and complete tetraplegia (C6 AIS A) left him with partial use of his arms and wrists and no active muscle movement from his chest down. Jason had excellent family support throughout his inpatient rehabilitation. His family had started making home modifications early on during his hospital stay, and as Jason's discharge approached, his mother and father were ready for him to come home.

Jason imagined walking out of the hospital at the end of his inpatient stay, not needing a wheelchair. Although he appreciated the work of his therapists, as his discharge date was imminent, he felt abandoned by his medical team. The dialogue below is an example of a typical conversation that occurs when patients express concern about treatment setting transitions.

JASON: "You think I'm ready to discharge home, but I can't take care of myself yet. I still need help zipping up my jeans and cathing in bed sometimes, among other things. My hands are just not where they should be."

OCCUPATIONAL THERAPIST (OT): "Jason I've been doing this job for 10 years. You have come so far here. Trust me in my experience."

JASON: "But how can I leave here if I can't dress myself fully?"

OT: "It is time for you to go home to your family. You will figure out the zipper, the cathing just takes some set up. You can do this. It is time for you to go home to your family."

JASON: "I feel like you are giving up on me and my recovery. How can I keep progressing if I am not in therapy every day?"

OT: "Your recovery isn't only about therapy. Remember how the doctor explained that recovery isn't dependent on therapy but on the time since your injury. You still have time to get more neurologic function back, and your hands will get stronger on their own with time."

JASON: "I won't keep making progress without therapy. I don't want to leave."

OT: "But Jason, it is time for you to move on. You have already been here longer than some of our patients."

JASON: "It hasn't been long enough for me. I am still making progress. I need to stay until I can walk again."

OT: "Jason, you have an AIS A injury, we don't know when or if you will be able to walk. You can't stay here while we wait for that."

JASON: "You guys just want to kick me out. I can't do this. You really don't listen or understand, do you?"

In this dialogue, you see the OT fall into the *expert trap*. The practitioner believes that the patient will feel their vote of confidence, when in reality the patient may feel silenced. The replies by the practitioner shut down the possibilities of a constructive conversation. The OT assumes that Jason will take their word as the final word and in one interaction change his mind about transitioning home. As seen in the example above, the patient became more rigid and fixed in his position, attempting to gain validation for his feelings and justify why he needed to remain in the inpatient setting. The OT has opportunities to affirm Jason's strengths and more specifically identify his goals but doesn't dive into them with these responses, resorting to an adamant, authoritative stance. With follow-up, utilizing MI skills, the OT could have gained an understanding of Jason's specific concerns about his transition of care.

Now let's see how with utilization of MI skills we can extract more from a single conversation and take a collaborative approach.

JASON: "You think I'm ready to discharge home, but I can't take care of myself yet. I still need help zipping up my jeans and cathing in bed sometimes, among other things. My hands are just not where they should be."

OT: "I hear you, and it sounds like you have some very specific goals you'd like to accomplish. Tell me your biggest concerns about going home." (Reflection, open-ended question)

JASON: "I just don't think I'm going to get any better without all the therapy here. I feel like you guys have given up on me, that I'm not progressing enough so you have to kick me out."

OT: "You have a strong desire to become independent with your self-cares, and that motivation has taken you so far here. These qualities won't just change when you go home. Are you OK if together we reflect how you and I saw yourself initially coming into our hospital and how we both see yourself now?" (Affirmation, asking permission)

JASON: "Sure I guess so."

OT: "Is it OK if I initially provide some of my impressions to you?" (Asking permission)

JASON: "That's OK with me."

OT: "Great and thanks. Think back on how you started to learn how to dress yourself. It took you 45 minutes to put on your pants; now it takes you 5 minutes. All you need help with is the zipper . . . and that is only sometimes! The last time we worked on this skill I don't remember you needing any help from me. How do you feel now about your ability to perform your morning routine? (Affirmation, open-ended question)

JASON: "I guess you did just stand there most of the last time we worked on dressing, and I do have a video on my phone of when we started. It took forever for me to thread one of my legs!"

OT: "So, you do see some progress in your program here. These are certainly positive changes that you've accomplished and noticed. Tell me about some ideas you have when you think about at-home solutions for getting ready for the day?" (Affirmation, open-ended question)

JASON: "Well, I'm having problems just with my zipper, so I think I will throw a key chain ring on it. And I figured out a way to get my electric toothbrush on by using the edge of the counter."

OT: "Excellent solution. You have been a great problem-solver from the start. What else concerns you about leaving inpatient?" (Affirmation, open-ended question)

JASON: "I did get dressing down pretty fast, but what about the electric stimulation to my hands that I get a couple times a week? And sometimes I have to call in nursing to get set up for cathing at night! I don't want to be a burden on my mom."

OT: "It's great you are thinking about your mom. She just told me the other day how proud she is of your progress and how excited she is to have you home. Given your fine problem-solving abilities, what are ways that you feel you can prepare for your evening, without having to rely on anyone else?" (Affirmation, open-ended question)

JASON: "Oh, well I guess I can set up everything within reach at bedside before I transfer, I remember you recommending that rolling cart for my supplies."

OT: "Jason you mentioned your other concern was that you would have trouble with the setup required for your electrical stimulation unit. Tell me more specifically what your concerns are with that if you wouldn't mind?" (Open-ended question)

JASON: "Well, I'm afraid we will forget where the placement of each electrode goes and the various settings. It would be helpful if we could take some short videos on my phone so that I could just show whoever is with me that. It could be easier to direct that way."

OT: "I think that is a great idea, and videos are quick and easy to reference for anyone. We can even video the basics of how to operate the NMES [neuromuscular electrical stimulation] unit. We've discussed some of the concerns you are having about going home. Can I ask you another question about home?" (Asking permission)

JASON: "Sure."

OT: "What are the things that excite you when you think about getting out of the hospital?" (Open-ended question)

JASON: "Just seeing my friends. Hey, my old manager just told me yesterday he's going to let me come back with part-time hours at the music store. Also, I plan to get back into classes in the fall semester."

OT: "All of those things are going to be so great for you to get back into. Your excitement is so great to see. Just because you are outside of the hospital doesn't mean your body won't continue to get stronger." (Affirmation)

JASON: "I know, this is just the beginning. I am actually pretty ready to get my time and my life back."

CASE 2

In distinction from the above clinical situation, the following is an example of a patient living independently who will now require a move to an assisted living facility. Judy had been living alone in her family home for 10 years since the death of her husband. She had three grown sons, two who lived locally and had been checking in on her often since her multiple sclerosis (MS) diagnosis 6 years ago. Judy was well known in her neighborhood. She took good care of herself and was seen regularly by neighbors taking her dog out to get her mail around 3 o'clock each day. In the last 3 months she had required three separate visits from emergency services after falls within her home. The young couple across the street began to contact Judy's children, expressing their concern for her living alone as they had had to call the ambulance for the last two visits when they didn't see Judy get her mail.

Judy was adamant that the best place for her was her family home; she had planned all her life to live there. A year prior she had compromised with her sons and agreed to have caregivers come in to assist her with light housework and meal preparation 2 hours twice a day. Although her adult children had expressed their concern numerous times, Judy was strongly opposed to moving into an assisted living community just 3 miles down the road.

In this case example we will first see how a clinician may enter a conversation about transition of care with judgment and preconceptions. In this short conversation, the patient's readiness for change is not evaluated, and the concerns of the patient remain unknown by the clinician.

PHYSICIAN: "Judy I'm so glad you came in today. I see from your records you've had three falls requiring hospital visits in the last 2 months. As a result, I've recommended a transition to assisted living for you, which I think will be a safer option given the progression of your multiple sclerosis and increased frequency of your falls."

JUDY: "Well, I'm fine right where I'm at doctor. I've got things to manage at home and have no desire to move anytime soon."

PHYSICIAN: "Your sons have reached out to me, and they have major concerns about your ability to stay at home. Don't their concerns bother you? I really don't want to see you put yourself at risk by staying at home."

JUDY: "My sons are overly concerned. They love me, but they are too cautious and they don't need to be."

PHYSICIAN: "Given your history, I think your sons' concerns may be valid. Can you see that?"

JUDY: "Well I've taken care of myself for many years . . . and everyone else. Thank you for your concern, but I'm not leaving."

PHYSICIAN: "Judy, I have seen other patients with similar situations to yours. Staying in your home alone can lead to detrimental effects. Are you concerned about what another fall may lead to?"

JUDY: "I am not the same as your other patients. Again, thank you for your concern, but I am going home now."

This interaction is directive and judgmental, with the physician attempting to use guilt to persuade Judy into moving when they feel their recommendations are not being followed.

Now let's see how the spirit and skills of MI, illustrating acceptance, collaboration, and empowerment, help differentially guide this conversation.

PHYSICIAN: "Hi Judy—welcome in, and please tell me about why you came to see us today."

JUDY: "Well I fell just a couple of times, and my sons are on my case about getting checked out. I think they are worried about me living alone. We both know my MS [multiple sclerosis] is only going to get worse, but I'm managing just fine where I am at. I want to remain living at home."

PHYSICIAN: "You have a good understanding of what it means to live with multiple sclerosis and have been managing your illness well for the last 6 years. You took the initiative to meet today; it's wonderful to see you taking charge of your medical care." (Affirmation)

JUDY: "Well I appreciate that; my sons think I have no control over any of this."

PHYSICIAN: "Tell me more about that." (Open-ended question)

JUDY: "Well they heard about my falls, and now they are convinced I'm no longer fit to care for myself or live alone, even with the caregivers coming in for 2 hours twice a day."

PHYSICIAN: "You sound like you are fairly concerned about your sons' opinions on your ability to be safe at home. Is that right? (Reflection)

JUDY: "Yes, I don't want them to be frustrated with me. I don't know what alternative there is. I've got too much to tend to at home. I don't know what alternative there would even be."

PHYSICIAN: "It sounds like your home responsibilities are concerning to you. What are the major tasks you are taking on yourself?" (Open-ended question)

JUDY: "I need to sort my mail every day, but most of all I need to watch after Hugo, my dog, with a.m./p.m. feedings and letting him out throughout the day."

PHYSICIAN: "You sound like you are an excellent dog owner and Hugo means a lot to you." (Affirmation)

JUDY: "Yes, Hugo has been like family to me after I lost my husband. The falls were scary; Hugo stayed by my side until emergency services showed up each time. I couldn't stand to leave him for some assisted living."

PHYSICIAN: "Is it OK if I ask some questions to better understand your concern for moving?" (Asking permission)

JUDY: "Well yes . . ."

PHYSICIAN: "It seems that the falls may have been traumatic for you and that taking care of your dog is your biggest reason not to move. Is that right?" (Reflection)

JUDY: "The falls were scary, and I am worried I'll just keep having more and more of them; but yes, mainly it's Hugo. I could never give him up."

PHYSICIAN: "What do you think the benefits of assisted living would be?" (Open-ended question)

JUDY: "Well I suppose I'd have more support, and EMS [emergency medical service] wouldn't have to break in each time I fall; but I can't give up my dog."

PHYSICIAN: "Hugo is a huge consideration when you consider a potential move. Your commitment and care for him are really noteworthy. What do you know about these facilities and their willingness to allow you to keep Hugo there?" (Affirmation and open-ended question)

JUDY: "I assumed they didn't, but I guess I don't know."

PHYSICIAN: "Actually, I know of a couple that do. Would it be OK if I gave you their names once I clear that with them? Maybe you and your sons could look into them and discuss different options. What are your thoughts and feelings on that?" (Open-ended question, asking permission)

JUDY: "I had no idea some allow pets. Yes, that would be fine with me."

In this example the physician has a much clearer understanding of Judy's concerns. The physician is aware that at the end of the discussion the patient may not be ready for change. As is often the case, life-altering transitions can require time and contemplation. He understands that he must increase his understanding of Judy's readiness to change and her unique contextual narrative. This conversation is more of a positive interpersonal interaction in which Judy's strengths are identified and her concerns are validated.

As seen in both of these examples, the use of MI skills can facilitate dialog, formation of a partnership, and exploration of the client's personal narrative and related concerns. In these examples, when MI skills are utilized, the patient felt understood, believed, and validated. This allowed a far more open conversation that was patient-centered and egalitarian in nature.

Conclusion

The nature of rehabilitation care is one that is surrounded by change. Patients are carried through these changes by their care team and often feel unprepared or out of control in the decisions that result in clinical transitions. We also see literature that supports the concept that transition of care is a specifically vulnerable time for patients and their families (Coleman, 2003; Le Berre et al., 2017; Miller & Rollnick, 2013). As rehabilitation professionals, we have a unique opportunity to help guide patients to a place of increased readiness for change.

We also may help to maintain patient-centered care by inviting the patient into conversations about these changes. Maintaining the spirit of MI in acceptance, compassion, and empowerment, we can support a patient's sense of autonomy during changing scenarios and care teams. Maintaining these qualities in the above examples demonstrated an improved outcome of care as well as an enhanced collaborative relationship. As clinicians, we can utilize MI skills via asking open-ended questions, vocalizing affirmations, offering reflective listening, and summarizing to guide our patients to a position of internal readiness and even eagerness for change.

Rehabilitation professionals may recognize challenges for patients within these transitions including momentum, relationships, resources, understanding, role conflicts, and coordination between care settings, which can impact the overall success and care of clients. We must recognize the impact these variables have on our patients and implement MI strategies for improving patient outcomes and autonomy through the ever-changing nature of the rehabilitation process. Although transitions of care are inevitable, they can be managed in a compassionate way that keeps the patient at the center of clinical decisions, thereby keeping the patient engaged and participative in their rehabilitative journey.

References

Coleman, E. A. (2003). Falling through the cracks: Challenges and opportunities for improving transitional care for persons with continuous complex care needs. *Journal of the American Geriatrics Society*, *51*(4), 549–555.

Josephson, S. A. (2016). Focusing on transitions of care: A change is here. *Neurology Clinical Practice*, *6*(2), 183–189.

Le Berre, M., Maimon, G., Sourial, N., Guériton, M., & Vedel, I. (2017). Impact of transitional care services for chronically ill older patients: A systematic evidence review. *Journal of the American Geriatrics Society*, *65*(7), 1597–1608. https://doi.org/10.1111/jgs.14828

Miller, W. R., & Rollnick, S. (2013). *Motivational interviewing: Helping people change* (3rd ed.). Guilford Press.

Miller, W. R., & Rollnick, S. (2023). *Motivational interviewing: Helping people change and grow*. Guilford Publications.

8   Anxiety and Depression
Charles H. Bombardier

Anxiety and Depression as a Challenge to Rehabilitation Engagement

Depression and anxiety are common comorbid conditions in disability populations. For example, the point prevalence of depressive disorders is 43% among people with traumatic brain injury (TBI; Scholten et al., 2016), 22% among people with spinal cord injury (SCI; Williams & Murray, 2015), and 24% for people with multiple sclerosis (MS; Marrie et al., 2015). Existing data suggest that 22% of people with MS (Marrie et al., 2015), 27% of those with SCI (Le & Dorstyn, 2016), and 36% of people with TBI (Scholten et al., 2016) have significant anxiety.

Despite the additional suffering and disability associated with comorbid depression and anxiety, mental health conditions tend to be undertreated (Bombardier et al., 2010; Cetin et al., 2007; Fann et al., 2011; Mohr et al., 2006). Limited patient motivation to undergo screening, reluctance to admit having mental health problems, passive or active refusal to accept referrals or treatment, and inadequate adherence to treatment are all potential contributors to undertreatment. Fortunately, research on depression treatment preference indicates they would be willing to accept some form of treatment (Fann et al., 2009, 2013). Nevertheless, these barriers to treatment also represent opportunities to use motivational interviewing (MI) strategies.

Charles H. Bombardier, *Anxiety and Depression* In: *Motivational Interviewing in Medical Rehabilitation*. Edited by: Nicole Schechter, Connie Jacocks, Lester Butt, and Stephen T. Wegener, Oxford University Press. © Oxford University Press 2024.
DOI: 10.1093/oso/9780197748268.003.0009

Using MI to Address This Challenge

MI concepts and strategies can play a role in accomplishing mental health screening, assessment, and treatment in the context of rehabilitation. One overarching strategy is to view this process in the context of the four foundational tasks: *engaging, focusing, eliciting,* and *planning.*

MI TO ENHANCE SCREENING AND ASSESSMENT

Psychological screening and assessment may be seen as unwelcome or stigmatizing by rehabilitation patients who may not be seeking psychological forms of help. They may feel threatened, scrutinized, or stressed by attention focused on their mental health. Common strategies for overcoming reluctance to undergo screening or assessments include *normalizing,* that is, explaining that it is part of standard care and that they are not being singled out. Similarly, it is useful to educate patients about high rates of comorbid anxiety and depression in people with their condition. For example, "As you probably know, it's pretty common for people with [your condition] to experience some depression or anxiety along with everything else. Therefore, we screen everybody for those symptoms." Further, clinicians may provide education about how untreated mental health conditions can interfere with rehabilitation progress and functional outcomes. In addition to or instead of these standard strategies, MI spirit and techniques can be used to guide the screening and assessment process.

Rather than beginning with a didactic approach or launching into screening questions immediately, the MI-informed clinician begins by engaging the patient. Engaging might begin with one or two broad, open questions to understand the patient's chief concerns before moving onto the clinician's agenda.

- "How do you think your overall rehabilitation is going?"
- "What, if any, concerns do you have?"
- "What progress are you seeing?"

Open questions activate the patient and give them the opportunity to share what is on their mind. Asking open questions and taking time to listen to the patient signals a different sort of relationship, one where the patient is an equal partner, not a passive recipient of expert information or direction. Open questions about the patient's chief concerns also give the provider the opportunity to demonstrate their knowledge about rehabilitation, empathy, a nonjudgmental attitude, and an approach to psychological factors that is measured and contextualized. In the end, we engage people in our areas of interest by meeting them halfway and first giving attention to their concerns and priorities.

Next, we begin the process of focusing by asking the patient for permission to discuss a topic. This can be in the form of a strategic open question or a menu of options.

- "Would you mind if we shifted to talking about how you have been coping with all of this?"
- "When you are ready, I'd like to get a sense of what you think is going well for you on an emotional level, what things are more challenging emotionally, and what we can do to support you as you go through rehabilitation."

Of course, it is critically important that if the patient expresses hesitancy about discussing psychological issues, their reluctance is met with a reflection that conveys compassion while keeping the door open to approach the topic at another time.

- "Right now, you are most concerned about being able to walk again and not that interested in talking with me about the emotional side of things."
- "You are someone who prefers to keep their feelings to themselves."

Once we show respect for the person's explicit or implicit preferences regarding psychological care, they almost never refuse the request for permission to bring up these issues with them again at another, more opportune time.

Presuming that the patient gives permission to proceed with the screening assessment, the clinician can move straightaway into standard questions. It is often helpful to demarcate a period of structured questioning as distinct from other segments of the clinical session. "For the next few minutes, I will be asking you a series of standard questions. After that, we will get back to talking about how the psychology team might support you through your rehabilitation program." Alternatively, if feasible and permissible, the screening process can be infused with MI-related strategies throughout, making the process more flexible and streamlined. For example, before asking screening questions, the clinician could ask an open question, such as "What are the main emotions that are coming up for you as you face this [disability or rehabilitation program]?" If the patient mentions sadness, the clinician can follow up with reflections and more focused questions that approximate or lead into questionnaires or diagnostic interviews within the depressive symptom domain. Once depression is fully assessed, the clinician can ask about other emotions or use brief screening questions from other domains such as generalized anxiety or post-traumatic stress disorder to ensure that other disorders are not missed.

MI strategies can be useful when difficulties arise in the context of screening and assessment. Sometimes patients flatly deny diagnoses of anxiety or depression when their presentation suggests otherwise. For example, a clinician might administer the Patient Health Questionnaire-9 (PHQ-9) to assess symptoms of probable major depression and summarize the results along the lines of "Your total score on this measure is 15, which indicates you have moderately severe depression." Patients might respond by saying "I am not depressed" or "Things are not that bad" or "Wouldn't you be depressed?" When this happens, the clinician has fallen into the *labeling trap*, that is, prematurely and unnecessarily sharing conclusions with which the patient may not agree. Research mostly in the field of substance use disorders has shown that it is not necessary or even beneficial for people to accept labels such as *alcoholic* or *depressed*. In fact, labeling patients can engender pushback from patients, as the examples above illustrate. To avoid the labeling trap, the clinician can simply reflect back the patient's responses: "You said you have lost interest in things you used to enjoy, are feeling down much of the time, are having difficulty sleeping, have lost your appetite for food, feel like a failure sometimes, and occasionally have thoughts of death. Did I get that right? Did I miss anything?" Reflections communicate empathy and acceptance. They also can promote greater awareness when the person hears back what they have said. Together they help set the stage for offering interventions designed to treat those symptoms.

MI TO INCREASE TREATMENT ACCEPTANCE

The next task is to foster acceptance of treatment among those with clinically significant symptoms. Traditionally, this task involves making recommendations or referrals to treatment based on the information gathered. However, we know that patients may not be ready to accept treatment and that simply giving information and recommendations can exacerbate that hesitance (Miller & Rollnick, 1991). Taking an MI perspective at this step in the treatment process means that the clinician will use strategic open questions to elicit from the patient reasons to engage in treatment as well as a commitment to do so. Empirical support for an MI approach to improve help-seeking comes from a randomized controlled trial in which maternal child health nurses used brief MI versus usual care to encourage women with postnatal depression and anxiety to seek mental health services (Holt et al., 2017). In this study the nurse (1) elicited the patient's story and how she was managing so that she felt heard, (2) elicited change talk using importance and confidence rulers, (3) provided information using the ask–offer–ask format, and (4) elicited commitment talk. The odds of seeking mental health assistance were four times greater among women in the MI condition relative to usual care. In addition, among those who sought help from a psychologist, 48% in the MI condition versus 20% in the usual care condition attended at least six sessions.

There are many ways MI principles and strategies can be used to facilitate treatment acceptance. First, we know that, despite endorsing mental health problems, patients may not be ready to accept treatment. Before even broaching the topic of treatment, consider eliciting or giving affirmations. Research has shown that having smokers write about things they were proud of before being exposed to anti-smoking media improved receptiveness to the images (Harris et al., 2007). Based on this principle, one could ask the patient what they have done already to cope with their anxiety or depression and use reflections to affirm their successes and underlying strengths. This line of questioning can build self-efficacy and reveal what sorts of mental health treatments the patient might prefer or be more skilled at. It may even be better simply to recognize and affirm the patient for global strengths or core values that have become apparent from the conversation thus far.

- "Before we get into the details of how things are going right now, could you give me a little background on yourself? What are some of the things that have been most meaningful to you in your life before all this? Some things you have done that you are most proud of?"
- "So you are a parent. You take that role very seriously and have worked hard at it. Despite all that has happened, you have kept in touch with your son, kept that relationship going, kept showing that you loved him no matter what."

If the clinician makes a habit of engineering opportunities to learn about things patients are most proud of or successful at early in the interview process, it will be easier to employ affirmations when appropriate.

MI strategies can be tailored to the patient's level of readiness. Patients who appear to be in precontemplation regarding treatment typically will not move into accepting treatment within a single session. Therefore, strategies that express acceptance, emphasize autonomy, and plant seeds may be indicated. The goal is to engage in watchful waiting, where the clinician monitors symptoms without active treatment.

- "You feel that you are already managing these symptoms well enough on your own. And to your credit, you are participating very well in therapies and making good progress. You really don't want assistance from a psychologist like me, at this time. Whether you allow me to assist you in any way is really up to you. Plus, you hardly know me and don't really know anything about how I could be of use to you. Would it be OK if we scheduled another meeting to see how you are doing? If these symptoms have resolved—great. If they haven't, we can discuss, and maybe at that time I can tell you a bit more about how I have worked with other people in your situation. What do you think?"

If the patient permits another meeting, the clinician can reassess symptom severity and provide feedback. If symptom severity is not significantly improved, the clinician may ask for permission to explain ways they have assisted other people in the patient's situation and provide a menu of treatment options.

When the patient seems to be in contemplation about engaging in treatment, it may be useful to identify the alternatives and engage in a process to weigh the pros and cons of those alternatives, often referred to as a *decisional balance exercise* in MI.

- "Right now, you are not sure you want any assistance with [the symptoms] that you are having. Would you be willing to take a few minutes to discuss the pros and cons of trying to handle this entirely on your own and the pros and cons of allowing someone like me to work together with you?"

If the person is willing and goes through with the exercise, it is important to end the exercise with an open question that does not imply an action, such as "What do you make of all this?" or "Where does this leave you?" or "What, if anything, would you like to take from what we just discussed?" The goal is to elicit commitment language, when the patient clearly states they want some form of assistance or treatment.

Next comes the planning task. During planning it is critical that the goals are negotiated, with the needs and preferences of the patient being accorded as much weight as possible. One way to enhance planning is to give patients choices. We know that choice improves adherence, and giving patients choice is consistent with the MI spirit of autonomy. There are several forms of evidence-informed treatments for depression or anxiety in rehabilitation populations and no evidence to suggest any form of treatment is superior to another (Bombardier et al., 2021; Peppel et al., 2020; Russell et al., 2020). Therefore, if the rehabilitation provider can provide patients with a menu of treatment options to choose from, acceptance of treatment should increase. For example, "There are a variety of ways to treat the symptoms you mentioned. They have all been shown to be helpful, and you can choose options that suit you." Describe the medical and psychological treatments available, and be sure to include "no treatment" as an option, to avoid triggering reactance.

MI TO IMPROVE TREATMENT OUTCOMES

There are at least three different ways MI can be used to enhance treatment: (1) MI prior to treatment, (2) MI as needed during treatment, and (3) MI used continuously throughout the treatment process. Brief MI interventions can be used prior to treatment to promote preparation for and engagement in treatment. A meta-analysis shows that pretreatment with one to four MI sessions improves the efficacy of cognitive behavioral therapy (CBT) across a wide range of anxiety disorder diagnoses (Marker & Norton, 2018). A notable pretreatment study compared four sessions of MI plus 11 sessions of CBT versus 15 sessions of CBT for severe generalized anxiety disorder (GAD) and reported that people in the MI + CBT group had approximately five times greater odds of no longer meeting criteria for GAD at 12 months (Westra et al., 2018). There were also less than half as many dropouts in the MI + CBT group relative to CBT alone (10% vs. 23%). Adjunctive MI treatment may improve outcomes of treatment for depression and anxiety by enhancing patient engagement in treatment (Romano & Peters, 2015) or through greater attunement to patient outcome expectations (Coyne et al., 2021), though more research is needed. Pretreatment with MI can increase the overall cost and burden of treatment and may not benefit everyone. Pretreatment MI may be indicated as part of standard care in settings where patient engagement is expected to be low. Alternatively, MI before treatment might be applied selectively for patients who demonstrate low treatment readiness during the intake process.

Another option is to utilize MI as needed throughout therapy to address waning engagement. One study that examined the use of MI as needed throughout transdiagnostic CBT for anxiety found that this approach improved both anxiety and depression outcomes relative to usual treatment without increasing the overall length of the treatment program (Marker et al., 2020). For example, a common scenario is that patients will participate in the cognitive elements of treatment but be hesitant to engage in the behavioral aspects such as graded exposure or behavioral activation. At this juncture, therapists are likely to feel the pull of the "fixing reflex" and want to argue for further change. "You have made such good progress so far . . . this is just the next step" or "How about if we just try a small experiment to see how it goes with you?"

From an MI perspective, we want to remain alert for signs of diminished engagement and resist the fixing reflex when this occurs. Rather, we want to express empathy and acceptance by reflecting the hesitance rather than trying to overcome it. When engagement wavers, it may be time to take a step back to explore what the barriers are at this particular juncture in treatment and (re)build motivation for the next task, if feasible.

- "Right now, you don't seem ready to try doing some of the things that you have enjoyed in the past. You have humored me by promising to try them and it does not seem to work out. It sounds like this is not the best way for you to get better right now and that we should pull back and consider what might be getting in the way or other options."

There are a host of factors that influence patients' preferences to stall or discontinue therapy, especially if they have responded partially to therapy and are suffering less. They are unlikely to fully appreciate the benefits of achieving symptom remission, and the likelihood of relapse or recurrence is greater given their specific constellation of risk factors (Bockting et al., 2015). This situation may present an opportunity to use an ask–offer–ask approach to sharing information.

- "You have done a lot of hard work changing unhelpful thinking patterns and are feeling better. One next step could be that you do some behavioral experiments to gradually get out there and do some of the things you have been avoiding. However, you said you are tired and have not been able to do any of the experiments the last couple of sessions." (Summary and affirmation)
- "Would it be OK with you to discuss whether to continue therapy now or not? The decision is yours, and I hope we can talk about it before you decide." (If OK, use an open question to elicit what they already know.)
- "From what you already know, what do you see as the benefits of finishing the therapy we had planned, including those behavioral experiments?"

The clinician reflects and summarizes all the reasons the patient can come up with. (If important reasons are missing, the clinician asks for permission to provide additional information.)

- "Is it OK for me to offer you some additional information about the benefits of sticking with the therapy plan to the end for people in your situation?" (Asking permission; if given, provide information)
- "Right now you are feeling better, and at the same time you are not back to your old self yet. For example, you are still reporting symptoms of [x, y, and z] on the PHQ-9. Research shows that completing treatment and getting to the point where you are feeling back to normal actually prevents depression from coming back. Otherwise, depression comes back in about 50%–90% of cases" (Zhang et al., 2018). (After providing information, the clinician elicits feedback from the patient.)

- "What do you make of the information that I gave you?" (Reflection and summarize change talk)
- "Where does this leave you with regard to finishing therapy?" (Attempt to elicit change talk or commitment language)

A third option is for evidence-based treatments to be infused with MI. One study that exemplifies this approach is a trial of CBT for major depression in TBI (Fann et al., 2015). In this study we planned to use MI techniques repeatedly throughout the sessions. For example, the therapist routinely used importance and confidence ratings to assess the person's readiness to engage in the homework assignments and to address expected ambivalence about completing these tasks. The therapist was trained to minimize didactic strategies and to use open questions to take a more eliciting approach to conversations around, for example, engaging in more pleasant or meaningful activities.

Many standard treatments can be didactic and directive. To infuse treatments with MI, whenever possible ask rather than tell. Rather than psychoeducation, use ask–offer–ask. A hallmark of MI is the notion that people will believe, remember, and act upon what they say more than what the clinician says. Moreover, we know that giving people information or advice risks generating resistance. From an MI perspective it is far better and safer for the therapist to elicit from the patient the notion that certain thoughts or activities contribute to their depressed mood or anxiety rather than teaching this content.

- "What do you already know about how what you do can affect your mood? What have you noticed?"
- "What, if anything, have you noticed about your thinking patterns when you are depressed?"
- "What are some of the situations where you felt down, and what stories do you tell yourself about those situations that make you feel bad?"

Then the therapist can selectively reflect the most helpful insights that emerge from the patient's responses.

- "Great point! You have noticed that whenever you make even a small mistake, you tell yourself that you are incompetent and worthless. Then you feel even more down and depressed."

Clinicians can infuse standard evidence-based psychotherapies with MI in several other ways. One is to give patients choices, for example, about which type of therapy to use, which therapy modules to use first, and what sort of homework to do. Completing homework is often difficult for patients. Therapists' expectations regarding manualized homework can be rigid and excessive. Rather than assigning homework, clinicians can negotiate homework and use MI strategies such as importance and confidence rulers to tailor the homework to the patient or make plans that are more feasible and likely to result in successful completion.

In summary, MI can be useful at several points in the process of addressing anxiety and depression, from promoting screening to enhancing treatment acceptance and improving treatment efficacy. Many of the suggestions in this chapter are based on extrapolations from related research, application of MI principles, or clinical experience. If MI is to take hold as a means of potentiating treatment for anxiety and depression, more research will be needed to support its application. Such research may be particularly important for people with disabilities who may have more biopsychosocial barriers to screening, accessing treatment, and achieving optimal treatment outcomes.

References

Bockting, C. L., Hollon, S. D., Jarrett, R. B., Kuyken, W., & Dobson, K. (2015). A lifetime approach to major depressive disorder: The contributions of psychological interventions in preventing relapse and recurrence. *Clinical Psychology Review, 41,* 16–26.

Bombardier, C. H., Azuero, C. B., Fann, J. R., Kautz, D. D., Richards, J. S., & Sabharwal, S. (2021). Management of mental health disorders, substance use disorders, and suicide in adults with spinal cord injury: Clinical practice guideline for healthcare providers. *Top Spinal Cord Injury Rehabilitation, 27*(2), 152–224.

Bombardier, C. H., Fann, J. R., Temkin, N. R., Esselman, P. C., Barber, J., & Dikmen, S. S. (2010). Rates of major depressive disorder and clinical outcomes following traumatic brain injury. *JAMA, 303*(19), 1938–1945.

Cetin, K., Johnson, K. L., Ehde, D. M., Kuehn, C. M., Amtmann, D., & Kraft, G. H. (2007). Antidepressant use in multiple sclerosis: Epidemiologic study of a large community sample. *Multiple Sclerosis, 13*(8), 1046–1053.

Coyne, A. E., Constantino, M. J., Gaines, A. N., Laws, H. B., Westra, H. A., & Antony, M. M. (2021). Association between therapist attunement to patient outcome expectation and worry reduction in two therapies for generalized anxiety disorder. *Journal of Counseling Psychology, 68*(2), 182–193.

Fann, J. R., Bombardier, C. H., Richards, J. S., Tate, D. G., Wilson, C. S., & Temkin, N. (2011). Depression after spinal cord injury: Comorbidities, mental health service use, and adequacy of treatment. *Archives of Physical Medicine and Rehabilitation, 92*(3), 352–360.

Fann, J. R., Bombardier, C. H., Vannoy, S., Dyer, J., Ludman, E., Dikmen, S., Marshall, K., Barber, J., & Temkin, N. (2015). Telephone and in-person cognitive behavioral therapy for major depression after traumatic brain injury: A randomized controlled trial. *Journal of Neurotrauma, 32*(1), 45–57.

Fann, J. R., Crane, D. A., Graves, D. E., Kalpakjian, C. Z., Tate, D. G., & Bombardier, C. H. (2013). Depression treatment preferences after acute traumatic spinal cord injury. *Archives of Physical Medicine and Rehabilitation, 94*(12), 2389–2395.

Fann, J. R., Jones, A. L., Dikmen, S. S., Temkin, N. R., Esselman, P. C., & Bombardier, C. H. (2009). Depression treatment preferences after traumatic brain injury. *Journal of Head Trauma Rehabilitation, 24*(4), 272–278.

Harris, P. R., Mayle, K., Mabbott, L., & Napper, L. (2007). Self-affirmation reduces smokers' defensiveness to graphic on-pack cigarette warning labels. *Health Psychology, 26*(4), 437–446.

Holt, C., Milgrom, J., & Gemmill, A. W. (2017). Improving help-seeking for postnatal depression and anxiety: A cluster randomised controlled trial of motivational interviewing. *Archives of Womens Mental Health, 20*(6), 791–801.

Le, J., & Dorstyn, D. (2016). Anxiety prevalence following spinal cord injury: A meta-analysis. *Spinal Cord, 54*(8), 570–578.

Marker, I., Corbett, B. E., Drummond, S. P. A., & Norton, P. J. (2020). Intermittent motivational interviewing and transdiagnostic CBT for anxiety: A randomized controlled trial. *Journal of Anxiety Disorders, 75*, Article 102276.

Marker, I., & Norton, P. J. (2018). The efficacy of incorporating motivational interviewing to cognitive behavior therapy for anxiety disorders: A review and meta-analysis. *Clinical Psychology Review, 62*, 1–10.

Marrie, R. A., Reingold, S., Cohen, J., Stuve, O., Trojano, M., Soelberg Sorenson, P., Cutter, G., & Reider, N. (2015). The incidence and prevalence of psychiatric disorders in multiple sclerosis: A systematic review. *Multiple Sclerosis, 21*(3), 305–317.

Miller, W., & Rollnick, S. (1991). *Motivational interviewing: Preparing people to change addictive behavior*. Guilford Press.

Mohr, D. C., Hart, S. L., Fonareva, I., & Tasch, E. S. (2006). Treatment of depression for patients with multiple sclerosis in neurology clinics. *Multiple Sclerosis, 12*(2), 204–208.

Peppel, L. D., Ribbers, G. M., & Heijenbrok-Kal, M. H. (2020). Pharmacological and non-pharmacological interventions for depression after moderate-to-severe traumatic brain injury: A systematic review and meta-analysis. *Journal of Neurotrauma, 37*(14), 1587–1596.

Romano, M., & Peters, L. (2015). Evaluating the mechanisms of change in motivational interviewing in the treatment of mental health problems: A review and meta-analysis. *Clinical Psychology Review, 38*, 1–12.

Russell, R. D., Black, L. J., Pham, N. M., & Begley, A. (2020). The effectiveness of emotional wellness programs on mental health outcomes for adults with multiple sclerosis: A systematic review and meta-analysis. *Multiple Sclerosis and Related Disorders, 44*, Article 102171.

Scholten, A. C., Haagsma, J. A., Cnossen, M. C., Olff, M., van Beeck, E. F., & Polinder, S. (2016). Prevalence of and risk factors for anxiety and depressive disorders after traumatic brain injury: A systematic review. *Journal of Neurotrauma, 33*(22), 1969–1994.

Westra, H. A., Constantino, M. J., & Antony, M. M. (2018). Integrating motivational interviewing with cognitive-behavioral therapy for severe generalized anxiety disorder: An allegiance-controlled randomized clinical trial. *Journal of Consulting and Clinical Psychology, 84*(9), 768–782.

Williams, R., & Murray, A. (2015). Prevalence of depression after spinal cord injury: A meta-analysis. *Archives of Physical Medicine & Rehabilitation, 96*(1), 133–140.

Zhang, Z., Zhang, L., Zhang, G., Jin, J., & Zheng, Z. (2018). The effect of CBT and its modifications for relapse prevention in major depressive disorder: A systematic review and meta-analysis. *BMC Psychiatry, 18*(1), Article 50.

9 Substance Use

Amanda Choflet and Jennifer Rikard

What Is Substance Use?

Substance use continues to present a major public health risk in the United States. According to the Substance Abuse and Mental Health Services Administration (SAMHSA; 2019), a staggering 60% of the US population over the age of 12 endorsed past-month substance use, including tobacco, alcohol, and illicit drugs. About 8% of the population met criteria for a substance use disorder, and only about 10% of those people received any kind of substance use treatment (US Department of Health and Human Services, 2016). Of the US population with diagnosed substance use disorders, the large majority of such disorders are alcohol-related (SAMHSA, 2019). Although substance use is rarely the presenting problem in a clinical setting, it is often a preexisting concern and therefore must be proactively screened and effectively addressed in every clinical environment. The prevalence of not only substance use disorder and dependency (SUD) but also risky substance use in primary care is understudied, though many report higher prevalence than in the general population perhaps due to SUD-related health problems (John et al. 2018).

While SUD, characterized by uncontrolled use of one or more substances despite harmful consequences, is an obvious problem in the rehabilitation setting, risky substance use, which includes any use of substances above recommended guidelines,

Amanda Choflet and Jennifer Rikard, *Substance Use* In: *Motivational Interviewing in Medical Rehabilitation*. Edited by: Nicole Schechter, Connie Jacocks, Lester Butt, and Stephen T. Wegener, Oxford University Press. © Oxford University Press 2024. DOI: 10.1093/oso/9780197748268.003.0010 is also of concern. Substance use is best understood along a continuum, with no use and no harm from substances at one end and fulminant substance use disorder with harmful consequences up to and including death at the other end. Along the continuum, people may engage in a range of substance use behaviors that result in increasingly harmful effects as substance use becomes more prevalent or relied upon as a coping mechanism (US Department of Health and Human Services, 2016). It is clear that substance use disorders follow a disease model of treatment and recovery, but there are often risky substance use behaviors that precede substance use dependence and addiction and may represent opportunities for intervention to prevent fulminant disease. Sometimes this is best understood using a non–substance use example, and one illustration of the relationship might be to consider the presence of colon polyps that often appear prior to progression to colon cancer. If the polyps are removed, it is often possible to prevent colon cancer.

Substance use is probably the most widely studied application of motivational interviewing (MI) techniques, and, in fact, MI was first described as a treatment approach as a result of unexpected positive outcomes in patients with substance use issues (Miller & Baca, 1983). While training counselors to deliver substance use interventions using client-centered approaches and behavioral self-control in 1980, researchers discovered that counselor empathy toward their clients actually predicted better outcomes than any other variable they tracked (Miller & Rose, 2009). From this work, a theoretical framework emerged describing the underpinnings of MI in practice, including a focus on eliciting change talk from the client and a focus on empathic, rather than confrontational, interventions by the counselor (Miller, 1983), which represented an alternative to traditional substance use counseling. In subsequent research utilizing these newly described techniques, MI was found to be effective in dramatically reducing risky drinking behaviors and, when combined with additional therapies, to enhance motivation to change and abstinence from substance use after treatment (Miller & Rose, 2009).

Challenges to Addressing Substance Use in the Rehabilitation Setting

MYTHS ABOUT SUBSTANCE USE

The tendency to overestimate the prevalence and amount of alcohol use serves to normalize behaviors that, in fact, may be both outside the norm and problematic for an individual. There is a body of literature that suggests that norms re-education, or correcting misperceptions of social norms around substance use, is an effective intervention in reducing use and associated harms. In the case of implementing substance use screening and interventions in clinical settings, it is important that providers avoid minimizing potential harms associated with patients' use of substances. At the same time, providers must be sensitive to any tendencies toward paternalism and instead approach the subject with a spirit of empathy and openness. Negative consequences can occur from subclinical levels of use. Identification and intervention work is indeed necessary, even sans a diagnosis of SUD.

PROVIDER BARRIERS

Often, substance use is considered an extraneous topic in many discipline-specific treatment areas such as rehabilitation medicine. Unless clinicians have sought out specific substance use training or specialize in substance use disorders, many lack training regarding substance use screening and treatment approaches, as well as a global understanding of the impact of risky substance use and substance use disorders on primary disease trajectories (Tetrault & Petrakis, 2017). As a result, many providers feel unprepared to ask their patients about substance use out of fear of alienating them or eliciting resistance and ultimately harming the clinician–patient relationship (McNeely et al., 2018). When they do discover substance use issues, there is a tendency to immediately "prescribe" abstinence or rely on an authoritarian approach to managing substance use behaviors (Henwood et al., 2014). MI diverges from the expert/medical model of care and requires that providers are versed in a different set of skills. In MI-guided substance use conversations, it is the patient's priorities around substance use that drive the treatment plan. The provider's role is one of empathy and reflective listening. These skills are enhanced by a team-based approach with consistent messaging by all team members engaged in patient care, which is sometimes challenging in the clinical environment. For this reason, robust communication and documentation by all team members are critical, and all team members need to be "on the same page" with an MI approach to substance use in order to facilitate change.

In addition to the lack of training and education related to substance use, many clinicians are intimidated by the perception of a lack of available substance use treatment resources or have been dissuaded from pursuing substance use screening out of an erroneous belief that leaving the questions unasked protects the practice from liability. Many providers are frustrated by these factors and unaware that their approach/characteristics can lead to negative outcomes.

PATIENT BARRIERS

Patients are in a particularly vulnerable position when deciding whether to disclose risky substance use or substance use disorders to their care team. They face what may be a well-founded fear of rejection by their treatment team, and many have experienced actual negative consequences and judgment by members of their clinical team (McNeely et al., 2018). There exists a power imbalance between the patient and the clinical team, with the patient often at their most vulnerable state. In the rehabilitation setting, patients may fear inadequate pain control should they disclose a history of, or current, risky substance use (Quinlan & Cox, 2017). This fear may be well founded as there is often poor awareness of evidence-based approaches to substance use harm reduction in clinical settings. Some substance use treatment programs require complete abstinence from substance use, which can make adherence very difficult for patients undergoing active therapy for additional comorbidities.

Understanding that people engage in the healthcare system as whole persons and not as a series of individual and distinct health issues, many may use substances as a coping mechanism and not have the benefit of alternative, more adaptive strategies. It is difficult to ask a person facing a serious health issue to abandon a coping mechanism during a vulnerable moment, even if it is ultimately harmful to their survival. Acute and chronic stress have been linked to substance use and relapse susceptibility via several theoretical pathways (Sinha, 2008). Patients may not understand the effect of harmful substance use on their overall health or prognosis and may not prioritize substance use treatment in the midst of competing health demands. Those needing treatment for substance use disorders may have difficulty accessing such due to inadequate health insurance, transportation difficulties, or a lack of programs that are geographically or temporally convenient or that are physically accessible for patients with special needs and co-occurring health conditions.

SYSTEM BARRIERS

Misperceptions around substance misuse, identification and treatment may add to the challenges of adequate screening in clinical environments (Table 9.1). Beliefs that it would require too much time may present barriers in settings that increasingly value efficiency, and this may be especially true for substance use issues that arise in the process of treating other, more tangible diseases.

Developing a rapport and helping patients to initiate behavior change related to substance use may take longer than a single clinic session and be difficult to measure in real time. Particularly if not addressed appropriately, the time frame for initiating behavior change with substance use may be longer than the time frame for the underlying course of treatment for primary disease/condition, again contributing to the difficulty of getting real-time feedback for effective interventions.

TABLE 9.1

Summary of Barriers and Potential Solutions

Barrier type	Example	Potential solution
Clinician	• SU not seen as important to specific disciplines • Fear of harming relationship with patient • Lack of training re: SU screening • MI requires abandoning the expert-driven model of care • Perception of a lack of treatment resources	• Ongoing, required clinician education re: MI and SU • Require competencies for MI in SU • Develop internal and external resources for SU referrals • Encourage peer support for developing MI spirit and skills; open dialogue regarding SU approaches
Patient	• Fear of rejection/stigma by team • Actual negative judgment by team • Fear of inadequate pain control • Use of substance as a coping mechanism • Lack of effective coping mechanisms • Lack of knowledge re: effect of SU on overall health/prognosis • Fear of provider demands for/ need for abstinence from SU • Lack of access to SU resources (for dependence) • Insurance/payment issues • Transportation • Lack of programs (systems issue as well) • Physical health conditions may limit available resources	• Implement universal SU screening for all patients • Ongoing, required clinician education re: MI and SU • Confidential referrals to SU resources, peer support, and medication-assisted therapy when appropriate • Referrals to mental health treatment to enhance coping in general • Providers well versed in myriad options for SU, with abstinence being only one • Equipping discharge planners with MI training as well as assistance to address barriers to treatment

(continued)

TABLE 9.1 *Continued*

Barrier type	Example	Potential solution
System	• Fear of liability • Lack of financial resources to support MI • Difficulty assessing efficacy of MI during episodic care • Lack of screening protocols in specialty care	• Work with IT to embed specific MI for SU documentation techniques • Build protocols for SBIRT billing

Note: IT = information technology; MI = motivational interviewing; SBIRT = screening, brief intervention, and referral to treatment; SU = substance use.

Many specialty settings lack proactive screening or treatment protocols for substance use outside of specific situations, such as preoperative care or the emergency department. Without proactive universal screening practices in place for substance use, clinicians may inadvertently contribute to negative stigma related to substance use by "norming" an assumption of abstinence from substance use. Some clinicians are actively discouraged from universal screening for substance use due to a perceived lack of organizational resources to treat any newly discovered substance use issues. Unfortunately, reactive approaches to substance use disorders ultimately require far more clinician and organizational resources than proactive approaches to substance misuse or substance use disorder.

SUBSTANCE USE IS A COMORBIDITY

Despite significant barriers from clinicians, patients, and the healthcare system, it is clear that substance use represents a meaningful comorbidity that must be addressed in order to resolve underlying health concerns and improve the holistic health of patients. Similar to other comorbidities such as hypertension and diabetes, substance use is often present even when it is not the presenting symptom and can negatively affect the patient's ability to recover from their underlying condition unless addressed (National Institute on Drug Abuse [NIDA], 2018). Compelling evidence suggests that substance use disorders and substance misuse contribute to negative outcomes in a variety of physical and mental health conditions (NIDA, 2018). Considering that the foundational definition of substance use disorder includes continued substance use despite harmful consequences, it is impossible to help a patient regain optimal function without addressing substance misuse or any lingering substance use disorders. While you may be successful in addressing an individual diagnosis, treating one disease and ignoring another is a little like changing the tire on a car that has no steering wheel.

How Can MI Support Substance Abuse Problems in Rehabilitation Settings?

MI TASKS, SPIRIT, AND SKILLS

Because MI was developed in the area of substance use treatment, there is a glut of literature describing its use in this population, so much so that it can be difficult to know where to start as an outsider to the discipline of substance use treatment. It is important to remember that incorporating MI spirit and skills into the clinical setting can reduce stigma and judgment by the clinician team even before a single patient has been seen because the MI spirit inverts the traditional approach to substance use management (Table 9.2). Typically, MI for substance use begins by developing rapport with the patient and building trust based on the patient's goals and needs. This is similar to the initiation of every clinician–patient engagement and fits extremely well with rehabilitation medicine.

Because MI incorporates a harm reduction approach that centers the patient's goals and needs, it can be difficult for some clinicians to "let go" of their preconceived ideas about patient adherence and morality as they relate to continued substance use. MI for substance use requires the clinician to accept their own limitations in directing the patient's behavior, which means that the patient may continue using alcohol and drugs in a harmful way during treatment for their comorbid conditions. Over time and with continued work, the hope is that the clinician will engage in MI-consistent behaviors and an MI spirit of empathy and acceptance that elicits change talk and, eventually, behavior change that results in decreased negative consequences from substance use. This task sometimes is short and sometimes takes an extended period of time, perhaps even more time than treatment for the presenting disease or injury. Some team members may be troubled by the idea of not "prescribing abstinence" during the treatment period, but the MI approach builds on the patient's own motivations toward reducing harm, encouraging them to build upon goal attainment. It is helpful to remember that empathy is a strategically important intervention. For most clients, the benefits of medical treatment, even with continued substance use, far outweigh the risks involved with taking a hard-line approach to substance use and withholding medical treatment.

TABLE 9.2

MI Spirit and Skills in Substance Use

Substance use example

MI spirit

Autonomy/acceptance	The patient's substance use belongs to them, and the decision to seek help or change substance use behaviors is theirs alone.
Collaboration/ partnership	Working together, providers and patients set individualized goals.
Empowerment	The role of the clinician is to elicit the patient's own feelings and thoughts about substance use and needed behavior changes, understanding that the patient already has what they need within them.
Empathy/compassion	Clinician empathy with the patient is likely one of the driving forces in creating conditions for change and movement toward goals. Empathizing with the patient is always the right choice, even if the decisions the patient makes diverge from the clinician's personal opinions. Empathy does not mean agreement.

MI skills

Open-ended questions	"Can you tell me about your drinking?"
Affirmations	"It seems like this has been a really difficult time. I'm impressed that you have been keeping up with all of your appointments."
Reflections	"You have been trying to cut back on your drinking and are not feeling supported by your friends."
Summaries	"So, you have been thinking about how much you drink every night and have wanted to cut back but are afraid that your friends won't hang out with you anymore. You are planning to talk to your best friend about your plan to cut back on drinking and brainstorm other activities the two of you can do together. We will check in again next week about how this is going. Does that sound right?"

SCREENING, BRIEF INTERVENTION, AND REFERRAL TO TREATMENT

One of the most widely used methods to employ MI in the clinical setting is the implementation of a screening, brief intervention, and referral to treatment (SBIRT) program. SBIRT involves training the multidisciplinary team in MI spirit and skills, incorporating validated screening tools into routine patient care practices, and using MI skills to initiate brief interventions to elicit patient change talk and behavior change. Several training guides have been developed to assist non-substance use clinical settings to initiate an SBIRT program in their clinical practice, such as the Centers for Disease Control and Prevention's *Planning and Implementing Screening and Brief Intervention for Risky Alcohol Use* (2014), the World Health Organization's *The ASSIST-Linked Brief Intervention for Hazardous and Harmful Substance Use* (Humeniuk et al., 2010), and the Massachusetts Department of Public Health SBIRT Screening Toolkit (2012). Because SBIRT is so well described and has been implemented in a variety of geographical regions, diagnostic settings, and patient populations (as discussed for primary care settings in Hargraves et al., 2017), it is sometimes the first exposure a new clinical team may have to MI principles, spirit, and skills. The reader is encouraged to explore these resources as a primer for deploying MI-consistent intervention programs.

Case Studies

CASE STUDY 1: "MR. PEACH"

Mr. Peach is a 62-year-old man with a new diagnosis of Stage 3a squamous cell carcinoma of the lung. He presents to the oncology clinic with progressive shortness of breath, weight loss, and a persistent cough. During his initial clinic appointment, which he attended with his wife, he mentions that he normally drinks "a couple beers and a drink," which the nurse notes in his medical record. During his intake appointment, nurse Amy asks to speak with Mr. Peach alone for a few minutes to discuss his upcoming treatment details.

During their conversation, nurse Amy focuses on building their therapeutic bond by employing open-ended questions and reflections with Mr. Peach. They discuss the positive and negative aspects of his alcohol use, and during the course of their open communication, Mr. Peach discloses much higher consumption levels than initially reported, including past signs and symptoms of withdrawal when not drinking. He tells nurse Amy that his true alcohol intake is about 80 ounces of malt liquor and a fifth of whiskey per day, or about 26.3 standard drinks per day. Nurse Amy knows that this amount of alcohol represents an acute threat to Mr. Peach's life should he suddenly stop drinking and, simultaneously, that Mr. Peach needs to cut back on his alcohol consumption as quickly as possible in order to start cancer treatment for his treatable lung cancer.

Nurse Amy and Mr. Peach discuss the pluses and minuses of his continued use of alcohol during treatment. Nurse Amy talks to Mr. Peach about the potential for harm to his cancer treatment and shares that she is worried that if he continues to use alcohol at his current rate, his treatment won't work as well or he could be in danger of accidental alcohol withdrawal if he is physically unable to maintain his current intake. Mr. Peach tells nurse Amy that he wants to quit drinking but doesn't know how. Nurse Amy calls the psychiatric liaison nurse and the social worker assigned to Mr. Peach, but neither are available on campus. She then calls the inpatient detoxification unit at the hospital, who refer her to two outpatient programs; but there are no openings at any of the alcohol treatment centers.

Faced with several "less good" options, nurse Amy and Mr. Peach decide to do the best they can with the resources on hand. Nurse Amy talks to Mr. Peach about the idea of weaning off of alcohol by following a schedule where he would drink one or two fewer alcoholic units per day over the next 3 weeks to try to minimize his alcohol intake as much as possible as his cancer treatment was starting. Working together, they develop a weaning calendar that Mr. Peach believes to be reasonable. Mr. Peach leaves with his wife, calendar in hand, with a plan to return to meet with nurse Amy in 1 week to review his progress.

Working together, nurse Amy and Mr. Peach successfully reduced his alcohol intake to two alcohol units per day by the time he began cancer treatment. He suffered no signs of alcohol withdrawal and was able to avoid any emergency department or inpatient visits throughout his cancer treatment. At the end of his cancer treatment, Mr. Peach told nurse Amy that their relationship and her honest feedback about her concerns were instrumental in helping him decide to reduce his alcohol consumption.

Case Study 1: Transcript

NURSE AMY (A): "Mr. Peach, I'm so glad you brought up your alcohol use earlier as we were getting to know each other. We'll be seeing a lot of each other in the next few months, and I want to make sure I have an understanding of your eating and drinking habits so we can get you through treatment as easily as possible. Tell me a little more about your drinking?" (Open-ended question)

MR. PEACH (P): "Well, I don't think I drink that much. It's just that ever since I lost my job a few years ago I've been spending time with my cousin Joey, and we just sit on the stoop and make trouble all day. I usually have a bottle of Jack [whiskey] with me, and I notice that I usually have to get a new bottle every day."

A: "You drink from the bottle throughout the day. What other things are you drinking during the day as well?" (Open-ended question)

P: "I usually have a couple of 40s but not until after dark when my wife gets home from work. By then Joey goes home, and I try not to drink any more Jack."

A: "OK, a couple of 40s. What is in those 40s? Regular beer, something else?" (Open-ended question to clarify)

P: "I like malt better than beer, so it's usually my Colt 45."

A: "It's hard to even remember the last time you didn't drink during the day." (Reflection/overshooting)

P: "I sure can. I got the flu and had to stay in bed for a whole week. I was sick with chills and fever the first couple of days, and then on the third day, my whole body started shaking like crazy. My temperature had been just a little high, and then it got up to 102, and my wife says I was out of my mind. She called the ambulance, and they brought me into the emergency room and gave me a big bag of bright yellow fluids. They wanted to send me to some kind of facility to get the alcohol out of my body, but they couldn't find a place that would take me."

A: "What happened after that?" (Open-ended question)

P: "After a couple of days, they sent me home and told me to drink lots of water and try not to drink any beer or Jack anymore."

A: "That was very frightening." (Reflection)

P: "Oh, it was. I tried to lay off drinking for a while, but Joey kept calling me, and I didn't have anything to do all day when my wife was at work. I cut back for a while, but then, after a few months, I was back to needing a new bottle of Jack almost every day."

A: "It must have taken a lot of willpower to cut back for even a few months. I think that's impressive." (Affirmation)

P: "It'd be more impressive if I stayed off. I know I need to cut back, and I'm scared to death I'm going to die of this cancer if I don't."

A: "Tell me some of the good things about your drinking?" (Open-ended question)

P: "Well, the good thing is that I like my cousin Joey, and hanging with him all day sometimes helps me forget I haven't had a good job in years."

A: "And the not-so-good things?" (Open-ended question)

P: "The not-so-good thing is that it makes my wife so mad. I also hate being afraid of getting that sick again if I stop or have to stop drinking."

A: "On the one hand, you like spending time with Joey, and it's been really hard to think about not having a job, and it seems like drinking helps with those things. On the other hand, drinking causes a lot of stress with your wife, and it's really scary to think about getting sick again if you don't drink." (Double-sided reflection)

P: "That sounds right."

A: "What is your understanding of how drinking affects your cancer and your treatment?"

P: "I don't know much about that, but I have been wondering. I'm a little worried that it probably doesn't help it."

A: "Well, Mr. Peach, I share your concern about how drinking could affect your cancer treatment, and I can tell you more about that, with your permission. You are smart to think about what might happen if you are forced to stop drinking all of a sudden."

(Affirmation) "It could be dangerous if you stop drinking suddenly and may be safer to try to cut back slowly so that you wouldn't get sick again. I care about you, and I want this to be as safe as possible, and I want to see us treat your cancer in the best way. (Empathy)

p: "How do we do that? I think I want to try to figure out how to cut back."

CASE STUDY 2: "ALICIA"

Alicia is a 35-year-old woman with a new spinal cord injury at T6. On intake paperwork, she endorsed "weekend" use of alcohol and illicit drugs. During a routine psychiatric consult, Dr. Serrano, a psychologist, assessed Alicia using an MI approach. During their conversation, Alicia talked about her weekend trips with friends to local bars and house parties, where many in her social group would binge drink and use both prescription and illicit drugs when they were out. She's noticed that over the last several months it's taking more alcohol for her to feel "buzzed," and she's taking other substances more routinely to counteract the effects of alcohol. She's noticed more acute effects of intoxication she had not previously been aware of (night sweats, head cloudiness, etc.). She's also started to have urges to drink even when she's alone and on days when she previously would have avoided alcohol. Dr. Serrano engages in MI-consistent dialogue with Alicia and reviews recommendations regarding substance use intake and the continuum model of progressive substance use. After meeting with Dr. Serrano, Alicia discussed methods for tracking her urges and set some goals for decreasing her substance use. Dr. Serrano and Alicia plan to check in weekly to review progress and work toward developing additional coping strategies.

Case Study 2: Transcript

Dr. Serrano (S): "Alicia, tell me a little about your drinking?" (Open-ended question)

ALICIA (A): "Yeah. I just drink on the weekends. It's a social thing. I'm a social drinker."

s: "You drink with friends on the weekends." (Reflection)

A: "Yeah, it's what we do together. Normal stuff."

s: "You get together, say, on Friday, Saturday, Sunday to have some drinks." (Reflection)

A: "Right. And we do trivia on Thursday nights."

s: "What about Mondays?" (Open-ended question)

A: "Yes, now that it's the football season, we do Monday Night Football. It helps to start the week off right."

s: "And Tuesday and Wednesday?"

A: "Nothing then. I just focus on work and go to the gym."

S: "What's a typical amount you drink on a Monday when you watch football?" (Open-ended question)

A: "Usually two or three beers. I don't go hard like I do on the weekends. It's relaxed."

S: "Monday drinking is pretty different than the other nights." (Reflection)

A: "Yes."

S: "The other nights you'd be looking to feel the effects, to feel drunk." (Reflection)

A: "For sure. I don't really like the taste of alcohol, so I just do shots to feel drunk faster."

S: "Help me understand. How many drinks does it take to feel the effects?" (Open-ended question)

A: "It takes around three to start feeling it."

S: "It takes quite a bit." (Reflection)

A: "It does now. More now than when I started drinking after high school. At first, I started to feel it after just a drink."

S: "You've noticed some tolerance, meaning you need more to feel the same effects as before." (Reflection) "Through the course of your night out with friends, how many shots would you say you usually end up having?" (Open-ended question)

A: "Probably about six, and I'm done."

S: "You're done." (Reflection)

A: "Well, no. I'm done with drinking and ready to switch gears. If I was home, I would pass out, but I usually want to take a bump to keep dancing or whatever we are doing."

S: "A little cocaine keeps you going instead of passing out." (Reflection)

A: "Exactly. My friends and I do it. Then after a couple of hours we all go home and get some rest."

S: "How is your sleep, and how is waking up for you?" (Open-ended question)

A: "It sucks. Sometimes I toss and turn and even wake up sweating. It's not great sleep. But it's what we do. It's overall so fun, and you just take the bad with the good."

S: "You enjoy parts of these nights, and it seems normal, but it would be better if you didn't have to wake up groggy and if you felt more rested." (Reflection)

A: "Yeah, and also I feel really nervous and worried the next day. I hate that. I always realize I spent too much money and did who knows what."

S: "You feel pretty awful. Not just physically, but you don't feel like yourself in your head." (Reflection)

A: "Yes! It feels like it will never stop. I take some aspirin and try to watch TV and distract myself. Sometimes I fall back to sleep."

S: "You have to try pretty hard to feel better after nights like these." (Reflection)

A: "Yes. I wonder if other people have these thoughts too, but I figure it's just part of it."

s: "Your social group is doing it this way, and it's taking a toll on you; but it feels kind of normal, so you keep going. You're not sure if there's a different way. You're also not sure you can keep going like this. That's a really tough place to be." (Summary/Reflection)

A: (tearful) "I don't even know."

s: "It's almost impossible to know how to enjoy your friends and not feel so awful after, not spend so much money." (Amplified reflection)

A: "No, I know how. Not do coke. But after a bunch of shots, that's all I want to do."

s: "You have a really good sense of how much it would help if you avoided the coke. And you understand the direct connection that using it has to the amount you drink." (Affirmation) "What do you make of that? (Open-ended question)

A: "I'm thinking if I actually drink beer or something, it would slow me down. I wouldn't get so drunk so fast."

s: "You're thinking that you could change the whole chain of events by starting off more slowly. Drinking beer and avoiding hard alcohol." (Reflection)

A: "Yeah, like on Mondays. Nothing bad happens."

s: "You know yourself well, and you have quite a bit of experience with enjoying your friends without having the negative things that come after it." (Affirmation)

A: "I guess so. It wasn't always like this."

s: "How important would you say it is to you to make a change like you talked about?" (Open-ended question)

A: "Since my injury, I have been drinking more, trying to get the most out of life. At the same time, I don't want to spend any more time in pain or feeling bad."

s: "You want to enjoy yourself and not make yourself feel sick or anxious in the process. That sounds pretty important." (Reflection)

A: "Really important."

s: "You're thinking you will do this right away." (Reflection)

A: "Yeah, no more of that. I'll do it this weekend. Beer for me. And not the strong, craft beer. Just regular."

s: "You're planning for enjoying socializing with your friends and getting rid of the parts you really don't like. How might this adjustment land with your friends" (Reflection; Open-ended question)

A: "Well I'd have to let them know what I'm doing."

s: "You would tell them, maybe even ahead of time, that you have this plan so they can support you." (Reflection)

A: "Yes. I think they'll be fine with it, especially if I tell them why. They've been supportive of what I needed to do for my recovery from my injury."

s: "You've seen that they want the best for your health, and this may be another way they can support your movement toward health." (Reflection)

a: "Yes, I think that's right."

References

Centers for Disease Control and Prevention. (2014). *Planning and implementing screening and brief intervention for risky alcohol use: A step-by-step guide for primary care practices.*

Hargraves, D., White, C., Frederick, R., Cinibulk, M., Peters, M., Young, A., & Elder, N. (2017). Implementing SBIRT (screening, brief intervention and referral to treatment) in primary care: Lessons learned from a multi-practice evaluation portfolio. *Public Health Review, 38,* Article 31.

Henwood, B., Padgett, D., & Tiderington, E. (2014). Provider views of harm reduction versus abstinence policies within homeless services for dually diagnosed adults. *The Journal of Behavioral Health Services & Research, 41*(1), 80–89.

Humeniuk, R., Henry-Edwards, S., Ali, R., Poznyak, V., & Monteiro, M. G. (2010). *The ASSIST-linked brief intervention for hazardous and harmful substance use: A manual for use in primary care*. World Health Organization.

John, W., Zhu, H., Mannelli, P., Schwartz, R., Subramaniam, G., & Wu, L. (2018). Prevalence, patterns, and correlates of multiple substance use disorders among adult primary care patients. *Drug & Alcohol Dependence, 187,* 79–87.

Massachusetts Department of Public Health. (2012, June). *SBIRT: A step-by-step clinician guide.* https://files.hria.org/files/SA3522.pdf

McNeely, J., Kumar, P., Rieckmann, T., Sedlander, E., Farkas, S., Chollak, C., Kannry, J., Vega, A., Waite, E., Peccoralo, L., Rosenthal, R., McCarty, D., & Rotrosen, J. (2018). Barriers and facilitators affecting the implementation of substance use screening in primary care clinics: A qualitative study of patients, providers, and staff. *Addiction Science & Clinical Practice, 13*(1), Article 8.

Miller, W. (1983). Motivational interviewing with problem drinkers. *Behavioural Psychotherapy, 11,* 147–172.

Miller, W., & Baca, L. (1983). Two-year follow-up of bibliotherapy and therapist-directed controlled drinking training for problem drinkers. *Behavioral Therapy, 14,* 441–448.

Miller, W., & Rose, G. (2009). Toward a theory of motivational interviewing. *American Psychology, 64*(6), 527–537.

National Institute on Drug Abuse. (2018, August). *Comorbidity: Substance use disorders and other mental illnesses.* DrugFacts. https://nida.nih.gov/publications/research-reports/common-comorbidities-substance-use-disorders/introduction

Quinlan, J., & Cox, F. (2017). Acute pain management in patients with drug dependence syndrome. *Pain Reports, 2*(4), Article e611.

Sinha, R. (2008). Chronic stress, drug use, and vulnerability to addiction. *Annals of the New York Academy of Sciences, 1141,* 105–130.

Substance Abuse and Mental Health Services Administration. (2019). *Key substance use and mental health indicators in the United States: Results from the 2018 National Survey on Drug Use and Health*. Center for Behavioral Health Statistics and Quality. https://store.samhsa.gov/prod uct/key-substance-use-and-mental-health-indicators-in-the-united-states-results-from-the-2018-national-survey-on-Drug-Use-and-Health/PEP19-5068

Tetrault, J., & Petrakis, I. (2017). Partnering with psychiatry to close the education gap: An approach to the addiction epidemic. *Journal of General Internal Medicine, 32*(12), 1387–1389.

US Department of Health and Human Services. (2016). *Facing addiction in America: The surgeon general's report on alcohol, drugs, and health*.

10 Cognitive Impairment
Connie Jacocks and Kristen Mascareñas Wendling

Cognitive Impairment in the Rehabilitation Setting

Clinicians in a rehabilitation setting often work with individuals with cognitive impairment and/or neurobehavioral challenges. Cognitive impairment may be an individual's primary presenting issue or comorbid with other rehabilitation diagnoses. Further, cognitive difficulties may be due to premorbid neurodevelopmental challenges and/or a later acquired brain injury or illness such as stroke, dementia, neurodegenerative disease, cancer, or conditions such as multiple sclerosis. Cognitive impairment has also been noted in orthopedic populations (e.g., individuals recovering from hip replacement). Most importantly, cognitive impairments in attention, processing speed, memory, executive functions, and/or language can pose challenges to an individual's ability to engage in the rehabilitation process (Whyte et al., 2011).

Individuals with cognitive impairment experience poorer long-term psychosocial outcomes, greater emotional distress, and less successful community reintegration (Albrecht et al., 2020; Hart et al., 2019; Sendroy-Terrill et al., 2010). Cognitive impairment also increases the likelihood of reinjury (Bannon et al., 2021).

Additionally, neurobehavioral features such as impaired insight and awareness, agitation, impulsivity, perseveration, and amotivation can present barriers to engagement in rehabilitation. Clinicians often identify impaired insight and awareness as

Connie Jacocks and Kristen Mascareñas Wendling, *Cognitive Impairment* In: *Motivational Interviewing in Medical Rehabilitation.* Edited by: Nicole Schechter, Connie Jacocks, Lester Butt, and Stephen T. Wegener, Oxford University Press.
© Oxford University Press 2024. DOI: 10.1093/oso/9780197748268.003.0011

the most challenging variable in the rehabilitation process. At the core, cognitive impairment and neurobehavioral symptoms affect an individual's ability to successfully engage in interpersonal interactions. Specifically in the rehabilitation setting, these challenges make it more difficult to establish a collaborative dialogue between the clinician and patient following brain injury.

When intentionally adapted for use with individuals with cognitive and/or neurobehavioral impairment, motivational interviewing (MI) may foster readiness for participation and greater investment throughout the rehabilitation process. Therefore, the presence of cognitive impairment does not preclude the use of MI; rather, it may signal a greater need for a rehabilitation approach marked by its spirit and skills. An individual may be better able to build a trusting therapeutic alliance when their clinician is nonconfrontational and collaborative and promotes self-efficacy (Medley & Powell, 2010). With an established trusting therapeutic alliance, the clinician will be better able to help foster readiness for rehabilitation engagement, regardless of the cognitive and/or neurobehavioral impairment that is present (Hart & Evans, 2006; Mateer et al., 2005; Medley & Powell, 2010; Prigatano, 2005; Sherer et al., 2007). In fact, an equitable and trusting therapeutic alliance, the hallmark of MI, offers the best possible context within which to understand and formulate the relative influences of neurologic and psychosocial factors underpinning self-awareness and engagement difficulties (Medley & Powell, 2010). It is also important to note that while cognitive impairment exists within the identified patient, clinician-oriented factors and the way the clinician approaches the interaction can either hinder or facilitate MI utilization, patient engagement, and the collaborative process.

An individual's ability to meet the cognitive demands required of rehabilitation activities has a significant impact on their engagement, progress, and ultimate outcomes, specifically issues such as length of stay, reinjury, readmittance, and community reintegration (Diamond et al., 1996; Poynter et al., 2011).

When clinicians first set out to utilize principles of MI with individuals with cognitive impairment, there is often doubt, avoidance, and reluctance. Common questions which may arise include whether MI is an appropriate tool within such populations, how MI can be used for an individual who is potentially unaware of the internal process of ambivalence, and how MI can be used with those who are incapable of advanced cognitive reasoning, reflection, and abstraction. However, it is helpful in this instance to remember that we do not use MI *on* an individual (nor is it something we do *to* them); rather, it is a strategy we use *with* them. Ultimately the utilization of MI exists within our relationship and interactions with the patient. Within this framework, questions about the use of MI with individuals with cognitive impairment evolve to include how we can respect patient autonomy and promote collaboration and empowerment and how to successfully engage the treatment team, caregivers, and family when their loved one does not have the cognitive capacity to do so.

When considering the use of MI in individuals with cognitive impairment, a number of conceptual and somewhat existential questions may also arise which are useful to consider. These include discussions of capacity, ability to consent to treatment, and balancing factors such as supporting individual autonomy while ensuring health and safety. Thus, the use of MI is emphasized for building a therapeutic relationship but also as a philosophy of development for supporting growth in awareness, identity, agency, and autonomy.

Clinical research on the use of MI in individuals with cognitive impairment is extremely limited, with great opportunity for additional study. In individuals with traumatic brain injury, Ponsford et al. (2015) demonstrated that adapted cognitive behavioral therapy (CBT) protocols which included either MI or nondirective counseling demonstrated greater reductions in anxiety and depression and greater gains in psychosocial functioning compared to controls. A review of the literature pertaining to the use of MI as an adjunct to CBT for anxiety disorders, although not specific to rehabilitation groups, indicated that, although the research is preliminary and has limitations, integrating CBT with MI is feasible and has the potential to improve treatment initiation, engagement, and clinical outcomes (Randall & McNeil, 2017).

The chapter authors attempt to base concepts and discussion on foundations of MI principles and skills, and infuse the use of existing cognitive skills and strategies to meet the needs of this specific population. The overarching goal is to better facilitate patient engagement in MI-consistent rehabilitation, thereby promoting optimal patient outcomes. In general, the integration of MI with neurorehabilitation programs is fertile ground for future study, one that we are quite passionate about and hope that the torch will be carried forward by motivated researcher clinicians and scientists.

COGNITIVE IMPAIRMENT

The etiology of cognitive impairment in rehabilitation populations is often multifactorial in nature. Contributors include injury/illness factors, medications, mood symptoms, chronic pain, and fatigue. Significant emphasis is also placed on the individual who has sustained the injury or illness, over the injury characteristics themselves. An individualized approach is therefore imperative, one that MI facilitates.

A person with cognitive impairment:

- May have difficulty keeping up with conversation due to decreased processing speed, making it more difficult to comprehend and retain new information. Slowed processing speed also often affects other downstream cognitive domains, reducing overall efficiency.

- May have difficulty sustaining their attention during a therapy session and become easily distracted by external (e.g., noises) and/or internal (e.g., hunger, pain) distractions. They may have difficulty sustaining focus on a task or switching between multiple goals within session.

- May have difficulty understanding spoken language, making it more difficult to participate in conversation and/or following directions during therapy. They may also have difficulty verbally expressing their wants/needs/thoughts/opinions about their injury and rehabilitation. Impairments in language processing present challenges to extensively conversation-based or verbally mediated intervention.

- May not be able to recall new information related to their injury, rehabilitation team, goals, therapy exercises, compensatory strategies, and/or discharge plan. They may also have difficulty with prospective memory or proactively implementing tools and strategies when needed.

- May have difficulty with visual perceptual skills, impairing their ability to effectively process visual stimuli and navigate their environment.

- May have difficulty multitasking, shifting between tasks, anticipating potential challenges, learning from feedback, monitoring and modifying their own performance, exploring internal ambivalence, reasoning among multiple potential paths, or abstracting short-term or interim aims to larger overarching long-term goals. Further, aspects of executive dysfunction can also contribute to challenges in judgment, reasoning, and problem-solving, which are pillars of the MI process.

- May overestimate their physical and/or cognitive abilities due to impaired self-awareness, resulting in difficulties with realistic goal-setting.

- May have difficulty with initiation and motivation, leading to challenges with instigating tasks and task maintenance and completion.

NEUROBEHAVIORAL SYMPTOMS

A range of neurobehavioral symptoms also often accompany cognitive impairment due to acquired or traumatic brain injury. These may include impulsivity, agitation, disinhibition, neurogenic apathy, and lack of insight and awareness (in the most severe form, anosognosia). Each of these may have a unique impact on how the MI approach is adapted. A focus is placed on apathy, and reduced insight and awareness.

For the purposes of this chapter, the term *neurogenic apathy* refers to apathy due to injury pathology, as opposed to having a purely psychiatric etiology. This type of apathy may result from disruptions to the anterior cingulate and related pathways, ranges from mild apathy to abulia to akinetic mutism, and impacts cognitive, emotional, and behavioral concomitants of goal-directed behavior (Marin & Wilkosz, 2005; McAllister, 2000). Disruptions in frontal–subcortical circuitry also negatively impact reward circuitry, including judgments of (at a basic level) approach versus avoidance, risk versus reward, and reward sensitivity (Alexander et al., 1986; Kalivas & Barnes, 1993; Levy & Dubois, 2006; Mega & Cummings, 1994). The impact of apathy and reduced reward sensitivity on a person's ability to engage in problem-solving related to goal-setting is an intriguing concept, although outside the scope of this chapter. However, it is briefly considered in a case example below.

The majority of individuals with brain injuries in rehabilitation settings also have some degree of diminished self-awareness, which affects the individual's ability to engage fully in the rehabilitation process (Worthington & Wood, 2018). They have difficulty in goal-setting, predicting their performance, receiving feedback, and modifying their behavior to improve performance. Due to limited insight and awareness, they may be more apt to become defensive and resistant to intervention. A deft clinical hand is required when providing feedback, guiding intervention, maintaining rapport, and fostering a collaborative relationship.

While potential difficulties are plentiful, the goal of this chapter is for the reader to view these features as challenges but not barriers and as important patient-related factors that will help to inform and shape the use of MI in interactions with each individual.

How Can MI Support Rehabilitation With Individuals With Cognitive Impairment?

MI principles and skills can be adapted to use with individuals over the spectrum of cognitive ability with the clinician being open, compassionate, and comfortable with flexibly implementing skills; and accepting the process will not be linear. Below, we outline concrete tools that are helpful for the clinician in remaining aware of their own internal process, while also implementing an MI-consistent approach in the interaction with the client/patient (Table 10.1).

CLINICIAN SKILLS AND SELF-AWARENESS (IMPORTANCE OF MI SPIRIT)

Clinician concerns about working with individuals with cognitive impairment can influence the spirit of how they approach the therapeutic interaction, termed here

TABLE 10.1

Take-Home Points and Helpful Tools

Take-home points for the clinician

    Remain aware of own bias, judgments, pressures, and expectations

    Ground yourself in the MI spirit: acceptance, compassion, empowerment

    Emphasis on engagement

    Emphasize choice and autonomy, even within limits

    Roll with discard

    Slow pace, narrow goals

    Adapt activities to be structured, visual, and tangible

    Can be slightly more directive, but always with permission, after having established
       strong collaborative relationship

    Avoid fixing reflex

    Synthesize and summarize information

    Revisit earlier tasks when needed

Helpful tools

    White board, dry-erase markers

    Laptop/Word document

    Client's external memory strategy (e.g., planner)

    Visual scales

       Importance

       Confidence

       Independence

    Goal–plan–do review worksheet

    Goal attainment scaling worksheet (modified for patient's cognitive ability)

approach bias. With minimal, atypical, and/or absent patient input or interaction in the rehabilitation process, there may be more of an opportunity for clinicians to project their own beliefs, impressions, and goals onto the patient. Therefore, successful implementation of MI with this population relies in part on preparatory work completed by the clinician outside of the patient relationship.

To create a therapeutic alliance and facilitate active engagement in the rehabilitation process, clinicians may benefit from consistent self-reflection to become aware of and manage their own frustration, expectations, and internal biases. For example, what are our own assumptions about the individual and their injury (e.g., someone with extensive substance abuse history involved in a motor vehicle accident), what are our assumptions about the individual's ability to benefit from MI, what does it mean to "help" a patient, or what would a "successful" use of MI look like within

Mindful Approach Checklist (MAC)
- Internal Assessment
• Approach biases/assumptions
• Tension
• Frustration
• Apriori goals
• Role pressures
- Tools/Intervention
• Diaphragmatic breathing
• Brief meditation
• Other relaxation strategies

FIGURE 10.1 The Mindful Approach Checklist for Improving Clinician Self-Monitoring

a specific discipline when working with individuals with cognitive impairment? When left unchecked, these clinician-oriented factors may lead to clinician-driven rehabilitation (e.g., goals set by the clinician, acting as the expert, succumbing to the fixing reflex). Resisting the fixing reflex (i.e., the urge to steer our patients in a particular direction because we believe we know what is best) and utilizing skills such as asking for permission are helpful in countering these tendencies.

For the clinician, mastering awareness of their own internal biases and tendencies which may influence the engagement, interaction, and trajectory of their work with the patient is foundational. In some instances, adapting the MI skills themselves is not particularly required or challenging; rather, the most significant difficulty is the clinician maintaining an MI-consistent spirit in the face of resistance, or, to use the most updated MI terminology, sustain talk and discord (Miller & Rollnick, 2023). We propose the Mindful Approach Checklist or MAC (Figure 10.1), for quick reference prior to clinical interactions. The MAC includes an internal assessment of factors which may influence clinical work.

ADAPTING SKILLS AND STRATEGIES FOR PATIENT USE

MI Tasks

When discussing how MI skills can be helpful when working with individuals with cognitive impairment, it can be beneficial to review the principles, skills, and strategies on the MI tasks, as discussed in Miller and Rollnick (2023) and illustrated in Figure 10.2. The traditional four key tasks of MI are engaging, focusing, evoking, and planning, within which the communication skills of MI are applied (e.g., open-ended questions, affirmations, reflections, summaries [OARS]; asking permission, etc.). A review of MI tasks is also available in Chapter 3 of this text. While it is true that more advanced cognitive abilities are helpful as the complexity of discussion increases, simplifying is possible during all tasks. In this way, cognitive impairment

Engage	Focus	Evoke	Plan	Revisit
• ACE • OARS	• ACE • OARS • Building Insight • Agenda Mapping	• ACE • OARS • DARN • Explore Ambivalence • Develop Discrepancy • Avoid Sustain Talk • Scaling Questions	• ACE • OARS • DARN • CATS • Goal Setting • Path Mapping • SMART Goal-Setting • Goal Attainment Scaling (GAS)	• ACE • OARS • DARN • CATS • Re-Planning • Re-Evoking • Re-Focusing • Re-Engaging

FIGURE 10.2 Motivational Interviewing Tasks and Skills

ACE = acceptance, compassion, and empowerment; OARS = open-ended questions, affirmations, reflections, summaries; DARN = desire to change, ability to change, reasons to change, or need for change; CATS = commitment, activation, and taking steps; SMART = specific, measurable, attainable, realistic, and time-dependent.
Based on Miller and Rollnick (2013, 2023).

should not be viewed as a limiting factor in the progression of the working relationship through MI tasks.

Importance of Engagement

In using MI skills for work with individuals with cognitive impairment, emphasis is placed on initial rapport-building and establishing a sense of collaboration. Fostering this emotional connection and a sense of comfort in turn can improve an individual's openness and willingness to engage, even when experiencing lack of awareness or insight, defensiveness, or rejection of the therapeutic process. Frustration and defensiveness due to reduced awareness and insight require frequent rolling with resistance and discord and potentially falling back to the personal relationship established in early phases. In addition, an individual with severe memory impairment may require re-engagement at the start of each therapy session due to the ability to recall new information from one session to the next. Over time, an individual with memory impairment, even as severe as in post-traumatic amnesia, will procedurally learn to trust the clinician and better engage in the process through positive, familiar, repeated interactions.

The Fifth MI Task

Miller and Rollnick (2013, 2023) introduce the subject of *flexible revisiting* to emphasize that progress through the, then described as four key processes and now described as tasks, is not linear. There may be a need to revisit earlier tasks to implement change. However, when working with individuals with cognitive impairment, we suggest promoting this activity and referring to the act of revisiting as the *fifth MI task*.

Revisiting is a useful tool to employ often throughout a working relationship with several goals. First, revisiting plays an important role in allowing the clinician to roll with resistance, or roll with sustain talk and discord, particularly when met with reduced insight, defensiveness, and frustration. The clinician may need to revisit the engagement task in order to re-establish rapport and a working collaboration. Revisiting the focusing and evoking tasks allows the clinician to review the individual's earlier stated values, interests, and aims and provide additional repetitions of information for memory, recall, and consolidation. Revisiting the planning task allows for reorientation to the steps of a plan for change, monitoring progress, and summarizing future goals. As is important when implementing MI, it is important to approach discrepancies in an individual's actions and their prior stated goals with sensitivity. Avoiding the fixing reflex and an overly directive style is encouraged (Miller & Rollnick, 2023), instead exploring ambivalence and inconsistencies with a humble curiosity and desire to understand. Asking for permission to share an observation (of discrepancies) can be helpful in preserving a collaborative manner and planting seeds. Changes to goals or changing the interim steps to achieve an aim are viewed as a part of the process instead of failures.

As long as the foundation of engagement is preserved, working among the different tasks (notice, the change direction is not referred to as forward or backward) can provide valuable information and details, strengthen the therapeutic bond, and plant the seeds of behavior change and maintenance.

MI SKILLS

Open-Ended Questions

Facilitating discussion through use of open-ended questions is a key tenet of MI-consistent intervention. It serves to invite communication, guide discussion, explore ambivalence, and elicit change talk, among other things. However, when these questions are directed toward individuals with cognitive impairment, they are often met with brief responses, an inability to fully expand upon reasoning or reflect on personal experience. Therefore, providing support when answering open-ended questions or by asking more directive questions may be useful. A funnel-type approach is recommended, in which questions may start quite broad but then narrow depending on the degree of cognitive impairment. When the conversation would benefit from asking an open-ended question to get a better sense of the individual's insight or motivation, for example, it is recommended that the clinician first provide the individual an opportunity to answer the question independently. If the individual has difficulty responding independently, then it is recommended that the clinician ask permission to provide written choices.

Questioning may be so narrowed that they become yes/no questions. However, this should always be attempted after first asking permission. For example, "I'd like to ask you some specific questions about your therapy. Would that be OK?" Frequent simple reflections (below) can be useful for pacing discussion and ensuring comprehension. It is worth noting that even individuals with significant aphasia can benefit from MI-consistent intervention. Use of yes/no questions if appropriate (vs. open-ended questions), visual and/or written multiple-choice communication, visual supports, and involvement of key family members are helpful. In addition, a slow pace coupled with clinician creativity allows for generation of novel strategies and communication aids.

Clinical Example of the MI Challenge

The clinician's open-ended questions result in short answers that reflect Client A's impaired memory and decreased insight and awareness, resulting in overconfidence and overestimation of current abilities (e.g., Clinician: "What do you need to work on before going home?" Client A: "Nothing.").

Possible Adaptation

If a client is unable to generate a response to an open-ended question related to goal-setting, ask the client permission to provide written choices for goals. On a white board or in a blank Word document, write several concrete, patient-specific, contextually relevant goals: (1) walking, (2) my left arm, (3) remembering what I did during the day, (4) having a conversation with my wife. You can also collaboratively make a list of the client's motivators (e.g., Clinician: "Why does it matter that you improve/get out of the hospital?": (1) My son, (2) My dog, (3) My independence, (4) Finally sleep in my own bed). If the client chooses multiple options, you can then rank them in terms of importance.

Affirmations

Affirmations are meant to highlight an individual's strengths and provide recognition and reinforcement for their efforts. This is especially helpful when working with individuals with cognitive impairment who may easily feel overwhelmed, defeated, and defensive. Affirmations can also serve to strengthen rapport when confronting discord and to focus discussion. For example, highlighting an individual's love for their family and desire to provide can be a reminder of personal values and a transition to how they might apply those values toward the desired goals or behavior change. Affirmations can be used throughout conversation and/or at the start of every therapy session to focus the client.

Clinical Example of the MI Challenge

Client B has limited recall of previous sessions and becomes defensive when working with their clinician. They feel as though focus is placed only on their limitations despite repeated affirmations. Rapport and engagement are suffering because of Client B's memory impairment.

Possible Adaptation

Create a section in the client's rehabilitation planner called "My Strengths and Accomplishments." At the start of every session, review the client's strengths and accomplishments achieved in previous sessions. Add new affirmations throughout the session.

Reflections

Anecdotally, we have found that complex reflections may confuse those with cognitive impairment given their abstract nature and potentially lead to the person feeling misunderstood and demonstrating frustration and defensiveness (e.g., "That's not what I said!"). For this reason, beginning with simple reflections using the patient's language is suggested, before moving to more complex/abstract language use. Basic one-word reflections of underlying emotional tone can also be beneficial (e.g., "You're frustrated/mad/overwhelmed") and confirming for the person. These points are integral to implementing MI with any population but perhaps more so in working with individuals with cognitive impairment in order to provide responses that reflect one concept and are easily understood. This recommendation is also grounded in an implicit MI tenet: Fewer words are often better.

Clinical Example of MI Challenge

Client C is verbose and hard to redirect during therapy sessions. They can also be impulsive, with impaired attention and decreased insight and awareness. Client C says, "I waited in bed for an hour this morning before anyone came in to help me get up. I didn't get up even though I wanted to. I know I can just get up and walk. I don't need anyone to help me." You respond by offering a complex reflection: "On the one hand, you feel capable and physically independent. And on the other hand, you recognize and honor the safety precautions of the hospital." Your complex reflection provokes your client and heightens their frustration, resulting in an unproductive downward spiral. The client says, "No, I don't honor anything this hospital is doing to me. I'm a prisoner here."

Possible Adaptation
Try offering simple reflections, such as "You had to wait a long time in bed this morning" or "You are frustrated" or "You would like to have more independence." Write down your reflections on a white board as a way to support the client's attention and speed of processing. Use the written reflections to focus the client and to support the empowerment and evocation of their goals and motivation for change (Miller & Rollnick, 2023).

Summarizing

Summarizing is a core MI skill but may have greater utility in working with individuals with cognitive impairment. It is recommended that the patient first be allowed a chance to consolidate and communicate their thoughts about the session. This often gives the clinician insight into which concepts have been internalized and others that may need highlighting. For example, "Tell me your thoughts on the session today" can be beneficial. Speaking aloud about lessons and goals provides additional repetition and cognitive organization. This may be followed by an affirmation about their engagement in the session and the clinician asking for permission to provide additional input: "That's a nice summary, I can tell you were very focused today. Would it be alright if I add a few thoughts?" Then the clinician may provide their own summary, highlighting impressions and plan. It is suggested that a basic summary statement be repeated and recorded for the next session, simplifying conversation to no more than three take-home points or reflections. These points may again be reviewed at the beginning of the next session, to provide continuity and a starting point for ongoing discussion.

Clinical Example of MI Challenge:
Client D has difficulty comprehending complex conversation, expressing their thoughts, and recalling new verbal information. It is challenging for them to summarize an entire session due to the severity of their aphasia.

Possible Adaptation
Ask the client permission to make a written list of the main parts of today's therapy session. Write down several main parts of the session: (1) reviewed schedule,

(2) practiced family members' names (5/10 independently!), (3) planned weekend practice. Ask the client to point to the part of the session that was most impactful for them, then ask their permission to write a summary of the session in their planner.

Tips and Techniques for Additional Intervention

Adapting specific MI skills and tasks is helpful, including altering pace and scope of discussions and adding visual presentations of concepts or options.

PACE AND EXPECTATIONS

As mentioned previously, slowed speed of processing affects how quickly an individual can take in and comprehend information, as well as their ability to process or mentally manipulate information and in turn provide responses. Slowing the pace of conversation is imperative so that the individual is able to adequately understand the focus and task at hand and to respond appropriately. Simplifying language to key words and basic concepts can also aid in comprehension. Further, breaking a session goal into component parts (perhaps achieved over multiple sessions) is helpful. Notably, much of this work is done by the clinician either prior to session when a potential approach is developed or during session as they assess the patient's abilities and then try to match an ideal pace. Finally, providing a basic framework at the outset of the session in a collaborative manner can allow the patient to feel more comfortable in terms of the expectations and focus for discussion. If written, it also provides a visual cue which can be helpful for redirection to stay on task.

Given the potentially slower pace and more narrow focus of sessions, the clinician may need to ground themselves in the spirit of acceptance and modify their definition of "success." This is not, however, a lowering of expectations. Rather, the ideas around what constitutes "progress" are reframed. Small achievements provide a sense of pride and improve self-confidence, often thereby increasing engagement and ongoing motivation and investment. In turn, a foundation is forged for larger goal attainment and maintenance.

GOAL-SETTING

In addition to slowing the pace of discussion, narrower goal-setting is encouraged. For example, instead of the goal of independently filling a pill box, a smaller interim aim may be to pick one medication and understand its purpose, while also observing a caregiver fill the box. There are a number of existing tools to help with goal-setting and establishing a concrete, visual, and incremental path to attainment. This includes setting SMART goals (those that are specific, measurable, attainable, realistic, and time-dependent; Doran et al., 1981) and/or completing a goal–plan–do worksheet (first proposed by Ylvisaker et al., 1998). Further, goal attainment scaling (GAS) was first introduced by Kiresuk et al. (1994) as a means to evaluate treatment outcomes in mental health settings. However, it also offers a method for identifying specific subgoals and monitoring progress toward attainment and a way to structure a conversation and explore ambivalence around goal-setting, as discussed by Miller and Rollnick (2013). For individuals with cognitive impairment, it offers a way to visualize the stepping stones of progress and a concrete metric by which to reflect and monitor gains.

VISUALLY MEDIATED TASKS

The clinician may select visual strategies and tools to augment skills (OARS) and techniques. For example, the choosing a path (Figure 10.3) provides a visual representation of patient and therapist goals. When the patient is involved in the generation of possible goals and chooses the direction of the session (among available options), this can provide a sense of heightened control and autonomy. Notice the goals are not in list format, which suggests an order of importance. Rather, as the patient and therapist generate goals, they are placed in random circles, thus allowing the patient to pick the one of greater importance at any given time.

In general, many aspects of MI-based conversation including exploring ambivalence and planting seeds, which are usually thought of as very high-level activities, can be simplified in a way in which an individual with cognitive impairment is able to better grasp and manipulate in mind. Figure 10.4 offers an example of a

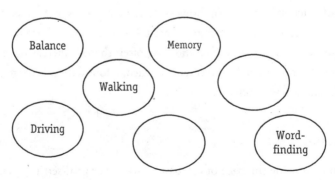

FIGURE 10.3 Example of Choosing a Path Exercise With Possible Patient Goals: "What would you like to work on today?"

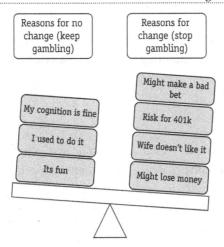

FIGURE 10.4 Example of a Visual Ambivalence Scale, in this Example for Exploring Gambling Risk. This Vignette is Further Explored Case Study 1.

"visual ambivalence" worksheet that could be used to visually brainstorm about pros, cons, and ambivalence. This allows the individual to "see" their thoughts on paper in an organized manner and raises awareness of internal conflict. The tilt of the scale may signify importance and readiness for change. A patient–therapist conversation around this tool is found in the script provided at the end of this chapter.

BUILDING AWARENESS

Three factors characterize effective interventions for promoting self-awareness and emotional adjustment: (1) a positive and accepting clinician–client relationship grounded in MI spirit, (2) collaborative goal-setting, and (3) selection of therapy tasks that are patient-centered (important to the individual, at their cognitive level, appropriately graded) and contextually relevant (appropriate to the individual's current context and life demands). The spirit and skills of MI are key in establishing this therapeutic milieu and accomplishing stated goals.

Primary components of building insight and self-awareness include predictions, self-reflections, and goal modification. Thus, when developing a goal using the SMART framework, a goal–plan–do worksheet, or GAS, it can be helpful to have the patient predict certain aspects of their performance (e.g., time to complete the task, percent accuracy). These predictions are recorded and, following completion of their task, compared to actual performance. Any discrepancies between predicted and actual performance are then used to modify goals moving forward. This practice of self-reflection, self-monitoring, and modifying performance is also excellent for building metacognitive aspects of executive abilities. Further, exploring factors which contributed to any discrepancies (e.g., distractors, pain, fatigue, loss of interest) can be a useful trouble-shooting and problem-solving activity.

Case Studies

Below are two case examples which demonstrate and integrate the spirit and some of the skills discussed in the chapter. This includes clinician-oriented skills at managing approach bias as well as intervention tools adapted for the individual needs of a patient with cognitive impairment. They provide some concrete, ready-to-use strategies for engagement.

CASE 1: "THE RISKS OF WALL STREET"

The patient is a 48-year-old, right hand–dominant, Caucasian male who experienced a left middle cerebral artery cerebrovascular accident (CVA) due to a left internal carotid artery dissection approximately 9 months ago. He completed 9 weeks of comprehensive inpatient neurorehabilitation and was discharged home with this wife. He continued to participate in multidisciplinary outpatient therapies. He continued to demonstrate anomic aphasia, right hemiparesis, and lack of insight and awareness, particularly with reduced appreciation for the impact of residual deficits on activities of daily living. He also exhibits significant neurogenic apathy and amotivation and cognitive rigidity. His overall functioning is consistent with Rancho Level VII: automatic, appropriate.

The rehabilitation team identified concerns about his continued day-trading and risk for financial loss. Concern was also voiced by his wife, who attended a majority of sessions. The clinician opens the conversation with broad, open-ended questions to assess his activity and insight.

CLINICIAN: "Tell me about your interests and hobbies right now?" (Open-ended question)
PATIENT: "Not much."
CLINICIAN: "What does a usual day look like for you?" (Open-ended question)
PATIENT: "I watch TV." (PT's wife adds that he has been trading again. He changed the password to the account, but she gets a notification that a trade has been made.)
CLINICIAN: "Tell me more about your trading." (Open-ended question)
PATIENT: "I used to do it all the time. Now I'm watching them. They are good. They are going up. I'm watching closely."

CLINICIAN: "You're very confident." (Reflection/affirmation). "Help me understand how you make decisions about buying and selling?" (Open-ended question)

PATIENT: "It's fine. . . . It's not risky." (Does not expand. Wife mentions he has access to retirement funds.)

CLINICIAN: "The team often recommends pausing/waiting before returning to activities like this after injury. What do you think about that?" (Open-ended question)

PATIENT: "I won't. I'm going to do it . . . right now. I'm going to keep doing it."

CLINICIAN: "You mentioned a recent task in speech therapy that was quite challenging. Tell me about that. How might that task relate to something like day trading?" (Open-ended question)

PATIENT: "It doesn't. . . . I would never do that task in real life."

CLINICIAN: "It doesn't appear to be very relevant at face value." (Reflection)

PATIENT: "Right."

CLINICIAN: "I'm curious, how do you decide what or when to buy and sell?" (Open-ended question)

PATIENT: "I don't know."

CLINICIAN: "I'm not a financial expert. Help me understand what goes into trading. What kind of thinking and memory skills are helpful?" (Rephrasing of open-ended question)

PATIENT: "I don't know, but I can do it. I am doing it right now."

CLINICIAN: "What is your understanding of how aphasia might impact your day trading abilities?" (Open-ended question)

PATIENT: "It doesn't. I'm doing it just like I did before."

It was apparent to the clinician that they were being met with significant resistance and discord, partly due to defensiveness but perhaps also due to injury-related cognitive factors. In an effort to roll with that resistance, the conversation was redirected to better understand the personal value of day trading, the personal enjoyment derived, and the current urgency about returning to the activity.

CLINICIAN: "You're quite experienced with trading." (Affirmation) "What kind of trading did you do prior to injury?" (Open-ended question)

PATIENT: "Changed job to trade but was planning on going back to work after a year because it wasn't panning out."

CLINICIAN: "It wasn't panning out." (Simple reflection)

PATIENT: "I wasn't making the money I expected."

CLINICIAN: "You left your job to try day trading, but in the end you weren't bringing home what you had hoped." (Complex reflection) "What makes you want to go back to it now? What is good about day trading?" (Open-ended question)

PATIENT: "It's fun. Potential to make money. Contribute to the family."

CLINICIAN: "Providing for them is important to you." (Affirmation/complex reflection). "What could be less good about trading right now?" (Open-ended question)

PATIENT: "Nothing, it's all good. I'm not hurting anyone."

CLINICIAN: "Tell me about the potential risks?" (Open-ended question)

PATIENT: "No, it's fine. I research the stocks and watch them closely. There's no risk."

CLINICIAN: "I have a few thoughts. Would it be alright if I shared them?" (Asking permission)

PATIENT: "Sure."

CLINICIAN: "You've talked about how much you enjoy trading, and it also gives you the opportunity to make money for your family, which you haven't been able to do since your injury. Providing for them is important to you. At the same time, you found it difficult to maintain prior to your injury. You left your job to try it, but it wasn't quite panning out. Your wife mentions worry about your retirement funds, and there is always inherent risk in stocks. It appears you have some mixed feelings about trading." (Summary of ambivalence)

PATIENT: "Yes, that's true. But I've always been the kind of person who doesn't like to be told they can't do something."

CLINICIAN: "Your team and family have concerns, but stopping trading would mean that you aren't truly independent." (Complex reflection)

PATIENT: "Yes, exactly."

CLINICIAN: "Let's try something different. Some might say that day trading includes inherent risk. Would it be alright if we assessed thinking skills in this area more before you got back to trading? I'm glad you're confident in your skills, and it would give the team a chance to see those skills as well."

PATIENT: "I'm fine talking about it more or doing more testing, but I'm not stopping. I'm going to do it now."

CLINICIAN: "Are there ways to minimize risk to your family as you get back to this hobby?"

PATIENT: "No. It's fine."

While the patient has acknowledged the concern of family and his rehabilitation team, he remains committed to this activity. In dialogue, it is evident that open-ended questions meant to elicit a clearer picture of the patient's insight and to build awareness have been largely unsuccessful. The patient remains entrenched in his desire to demonstrate his independence and autonomy by continuing this activity. He also continues to exhibit reduced insight into potential risks and the impact of his cognitive impairment on daily function. The session is nearing an end, and therefore the clinician decides to revisit the engagement phase, to allow for the possibility of ongoing discussion.

> CLINICIAN: "We're at an impasse here, and I'm not sure we will agree." (Stated with compassion and pragmatism)
>
> PATIENT: "True."
>
> CLINICIAN: "You're very passionate about this and confident in your skills." (Affirmation) "I can see that it's meaningful to you in terms of the enjoyment it provides and the opportunity to generate income for your family." (Complex reflection)
>
> PATIENT: "Absolutely."
>
> CLINICIAN: "I'd like the chance to learn more from you about trading. Would it be alright if we continued this discussion next time so I could better understand your passion about this?" (Asking permission with humble curiosity)
>
> PATIENT: "Yes, that's fine."
>
> CLINICIAN: "If not stopping altogether, do you think you could pause for just 1 week in trading so that we have time to further discuss?"
>
> PATIENT: "Fine. OK—that's fine."

This discussion demonstrates an alternative definition of a "successful" session or interaction. Success is not always a "win" but may be a "save," and preserving the collaborative relationship and rapport is of utmost importance. The patient has agreed to pause on this activity while allowing for further assessment by his rehabilitation team, which also allows additional time for discussion, building insight, and exploring ambivalence and behavior change. Key components of this discussion included the following:

1. Recognition of discord
2. Rolling with sustain talk and discord.
3. Use of open-ended questions to assess understanding, insight, and awareness
4. Use of affirmations and reflections to convey understanding and reduce defensiveness
5. Revisiting the engagement phase to maintain rapport

READER REFLECTION QUESTIONS

- What pressures might the clinician be experiencing?
- What expectations or goals might the clinician have, in addition to the team?

- What are the patient's goals?
- What skills did you observe?
- What might you add?
- What might you do differently?
- Where would you go next?

CASE 2: "THE SURPRISINGLY INSIGHTFUL PATIENT"

The patient is a 60-year-old, right hand–dominant, Caucasian male who experienced a traumatic brain injury after being struck in the head by a steel pulley at work approximately 4 months ago. As a result of the traumatic brain injury, he also had a right middle cerebral artery distribution subacute ischemic CVA. He has completed 2 months of inpatient rehabilitation, and he will be discharging to his sister's home in 1 month. His impairments include impaired attention, low frustration tolerance and task vigilance, disinhibition and often inappropriate behaviors and comments, severely impaired verbal memory, impaired problem-solving/reasoning, impaired insight/awareness, fluent aphasia, left neglect, left field cut, and left hemiplegia. He frequently confabulates (e.g., states that his semi-truck is parked down the road from the hospital) and has seemingly no awareness, per rehab team, of appropriate therapy goals. His stated goals are "to get out of the hospital," "to get back to normal," and "to lay down as much as possible." All of his impairments result in decreased engagement on rehabilitation goals and therapy tasks.

Prior to discharge, his rehabilitation team hopes to decrease caregiver burden as he currently requires two people for transfers and dressing and is completely depending on others to initiate activities throughout his day. Specific short-term goals include improving safety and efficiency of transfers, increasing independence with dressing, and increasing initiation of necessary (e.g., medication) and fun (e.g., TV, music) activities. The patient's occupational therapist (listed as "OT") reached out to his speech language pathologist (listed as "SLP") to help focus the patient (PT) on his rehab goals and increase engagement in OT sessions. After a brief introduction to orient the patient to the clinicians and the place, time, and purpose of co-treatment, the SLP starts by focusing the patient through use of ACE (acceptance, compassion, and empowerment), OARS, and insight-building. The clinician keeps the conversational pace slow and repeats key concepts and/or writes them on a white board.

SPEECH LANGUAGE PATHOLOGIST (SLP): "Would it be OK with you if we talk a little bit today to focus on what you're doing here in this hospital?" (Asking permission)
PATIENT: "OK, go ahead, talk a little bit! Not a lot! Just a little bit."

SLP: "How did your stroke impact your body?" (Open-ended question)

PATIENT: "It just about wiped me out. It hurt it pretty bad. Lost a lot of strength . . . a lot of my coordination, which affects everything else. Oddball stuff like that."

SLP: "So you notice it did impact your body. Strength, coordination, timing." (Simple reflection) "Going through your day, how does a loss of coordination impact you?" (Open-ended question)

PATIENT: "It affects you in how you eat your lunch, how you eat your breakfast. All your bowel movements . . . when you have to have a lava flow going to the bathroom . . . a lava flow or a urination. That kind of stuff."

SLP: "Before your stroke, you used to be able to go to the bathroom by yourself." (Simple reflection)

PATIENT: "Yeah."

SLP: "What's it like now to go to the bathroom?" (Open-ended question)

PATIENT: "It's like you need an army with all the people that need to go with you. You have to take 50,000 rolls of toilet paper."

SLP: "You need a lot more supplies and a lot more help." (Simple reflection)

PATIENT: "Yeah, yeah."

SLP: "Can I write these things down, the things you said your stroke has impacted?" (Asking permission)

PATIENT: "Yeah."

SLP: "You're a smart guy. Whenever we work together, you always have ideas about stuff you need to work on." (Affirmation) (The clinician writes "meals" and "going to the bathroom" on white board.) "So let's start at the beginning of your day. You wake up, you go to the bathroom with assistance, you eat breakfast with assistance. Then what happens?" (Open-ended question)

PATIENT: "You have to get dressed."

SLP: "How's that going right now, getting dressed?" (Open-ended question)

PATIENT: "You just seen that Lucy had to help me. I gotta get help to get dressed."

SLP: "Getting dressed now feels different than before your stroke." (Simple reflection)

PATIENT: "Yeah, I can't either lift them all or bend the right way. My body won't twist the right way or move the right way."

SLP: "You really are noticing that it's not just strength that's changed—it's coordination and sounds like flexibility too. You're on fire! You're talking like a therapist." (Simple reflection, affirmation)

PATIENT: "You better watch out. I'm gonna get your job! I want your job!"

SLP: "Strength. Coordination. Flexibility. OK, so far you have mentioned that your stroke has impacted the way you eat, the way you go the bathroom, and the way you get dressed." (Summary)

PATEINT: "Exactly."

Possible Patient Goals

<u>Possible Goals</u>

1. Meals

2. Going to the bathroom

3. Getting dressed

The clinician (speech language pathologist) and patient have now focused in on three broad goal areas: eating meals, going to the bathroom, and getting dressed. The clinician honors the patient's autonomy by asking him which goal he would like to focus on today. He said he did not care.

> SLP: "You're easy to work with! I get to choose? OK, well, let's ask your OT."
> OT: "Well, since you're cold all the time, let's talk about getting dressed."
> SLP: "Can we talk about how much help you need to get dressed right now?"
> PATIENT: "Sure."

The clinician moves to the "evoke" stage, and they start to explore the patient's motivation for improving his ability to get dressed. The patient is reminded that he will soon be discharging from the hospital and will be moving in with his sister, who will be his primary caregiver. The patient insightfully states that he wants to be able to do more by himself so that his sister doesn't have to help him as much. The clinician then uses a simplified version of GAS to better understand what improving his ability to get dressed would look like for specifically this patient.

> SLP: "How much help do you need to get dressed right now?" (Open-ended question)

Big Picture Goal

Goal	I want to have only 1 person help me get dressed (because that's how it's going to be once I go home)
Now	I need 2 people to help me get dressed
↓	At least I don't need 3 people to help me get dressed.

PATIENT: "Usually I need two girls plus myself. I guess I could do it with one, but it's not fast enough, so I cool off . . . get cold. Maybe I could get away with just one person. I don't know!"

SLP: "I like that. One thing you're saying is we gotta wait and see. There's no way we can predict the future. And another thing you're saying is maybe we could shoot for one person. That just one person helping you could be your goal." (Reflection)

PATIENT: "Yeah."

SLP: "How much more would you want to be able to help?" (Open-ended question)

PATIENT: "Maybe I could stand up, tuck stuff in, grab the next piece of clothes."

SLP: "You have some great ideas. You are a real team member." (Affirmation)

The clinician and patient focus in on the goal of getting dressed with only one person's support. With the OT's guidance, they then narrow in on him being able to bend over more in his wheelchair during dressing. This helps the patient focus in on what he could do to work on his goal of decreasing the amount of help he'll need from his session today during his OT session. A modified GAS is used to scale his long-term goal (i.e., dressing with one caregiver assisting) and short-term goal (i.e., bending over 60 degrees to assist more with dressing).

Handwritten depiction of modified goal attainment scaling during patient session.

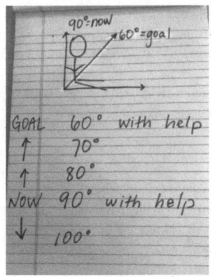

SLP: "To summarize our session, your main goal is to get dressed with the help of only one person." (Summary)

PATIENT: "Yep, that's right."

SLP: "And to work toward that goal, we are going to start by helping you lean forward more in your wheelchair. That way your sister can more easily pull your shirt down your back when she helps you get dressed. How does that sound?" (Summary)

PATIENT: "Sounds like a plan, Stan."

These goals, paired with their visual aids and the patient's verbalized motivation for change (i.e., decrease burden on sister), are revisited at the start of each session to help the patient re-engage, refocus, and replan, to maximize participation in therapy.

This discussion demonstrates that patients with cognitive impairment can show surprising levels of insight and awareness into their physical and cognitive impairments when given the opportunity and when paired with adequate support. This patient appropriately responded to open-ended questions about his current status, potential goal areas, and motivation for change. At face value, this patient appeared to be too confused and uninsightful to be able to actively participate in a meaningful and appropriate way. With realistic clinician expectations and open-mindedness going into the interaction, and with modified, flexible use of MI philosophy and tools, a lower-level inpatient with cognitive impairment is given the chance to more fully engage in his rehabilitation program and long-term outcomes.

Key components of this discussion included the following:

1. Focusing and redirecting while honoring patient autonomy
2. Keeping concepts and statements simple
3. Use of visual supports to support attention and verbal memory
4. Use of repetition and procedural memory by revisiting the main concepts from this conversation briefly at the beginning of each subsequent therapy session
5. MI philosophy and tools adapted to help lower-level patients with limited day-to-day memory engage in rehabilitation

READER REFLECTION QUESTIONS

- What pressures might the clinician be experiencing?
- What expectations or goals might the clinician have, in addition to the team?
- What are the patient's goals?
- What skills did you observe?
- What might you add?
- What might you do differently?
- Where would you go next?

Summary

Cognitive impairment and neurobehavioral challenges are prevalent across rehabilitation populations. Cognitive impairments (speed of processing, attention, memory, language skills, visuospatial processing, executive functions) and neurobehavioral challenges (impulsivity, agitation, apathy, reduced insight and awareness) affect engagement in rehabilitation and treatment, as well as psychosocial outcomes and community reintegration. A clinician can more effectively work with these patients by using MI-consistent strategies for self-monitoring and infusing the interaction with the MI spirit. Despite challenges, the MI spirit and skills can be infused throughout the rehabilitation process and modified to meet a patient's abilities. MI is perhaps best utilized when facilitating the growth, awareness, recovery, autonomy, and ultimate independence of individuals with cognitive impairment due to neurologic injury and illness.

References

Albrecht, J. S., Abariga, S. A., Rao, V., & Wickwire, E. M. (2020). Incidence of new neuropsychiatric disorder diagnoses following traumatic brain injury. *Journal of Head Trauma Rehabilitation, 35*(4), E352–E360.

Alexander, G. E., DeLong, M. R., & Strick, P. L. (1986). Parallel organization of functionally segregated circuits linking basal ganglia and cortex. *Annual Review of Neuroscience, 9*, 357–381.

Bannon, S. M., Kumar, R. G., Bogner, J., O'Neil-Pirozzi, T. M., Spielman, L., Watson, E. M., & Dams-O'Connor, K. (2021). Reinjury after moderate to severe TBI: Rates and risk factors in the NIDILRR traumatic brain injury model systems. *Journal of Head Trauma Rehabilitation, 36*(1), E50–E60.

Diamond, P. T., Felsenthal, G., Macciocchi, S. N., Butler, D. H., & Lally-Cassady, D. (1996). Effect of cognitive impairment on rehabilitation outcome. *American Journal of Physical Medicine & Rehabilitation, 75*(1), 40–43.

Doran, G. T., Miller, A., & Cunningham, J. (1981). There's a S.M.A.R.T. way to write management's goals and objectives. *Management Review, 70*(11), 35–36.

Hart, T., & Evans, J. (2006). Self-regulation and goal theories in brain injury rehabilitation. *Journal of Head Trauma Rehabilitation, 21*(2), 142–155.

Hart, T., Ketchum, J. M., O'Neil-Pirozzi, T. M., Novack, T. A., Johnson-Greene, D., & Dams-O'Connor, K. (2019). Neurocognitive status and return to work after moderate to severe traumatic brain injury. *Rehabilitation Psychology, 64*(4), 435–444.

Kalivas, P., & Barnes, C. (1993). *Limbic motor circuitry and neuropsychiatry.* CRC Press.

Kiresuk, T. J., Smith, A., & Cardillo, J. E. (Eds.). (1994). *Goal attainment scaling: Applications, theory, and measurement.* Lawrence Erlbaum Associates.

Levy, R., & Dubois, B. (2006). Apathy and the functional anatomy of the prefrontal cortex–basal ganglia circuits. *Cerebral Cortex, 16*, 916–928.

Marin, R. S., & Wilkosz, P. A. (2005). Disorders of diminished motivation. *Journal of Head Trauma Rehabilitation, 20*, 377–388.

Mateer, C. A., Sira, C. S., & O'Connell, M. A. (2005). Putting Humpty Dumpty together again: The importance of integrating cognitive and emotional interventions. *Journal of Head Trauma Rehabilitation, 20*(1), 62–75.

McAllister, T. W. (2000). Apathy. *Seminars in Clinical Neuropsychiatry, 5*, 275–282.

Medley, A. R., & Powell, T. (2010). Motivational interviewing to promote self-awareness and engagement in rehabilitation following acquired brain injury: A conceptual review. *Neuropsychological Rehabilitation, 20*(4), 481–508.

Mega, M. S., & Cummings, J. L. (1994). Frontal-subcortical circuits and neuropsychiatric disorders. *Journal of Neuropsychiatry and Clinical Neurosciences, 6*, 358–370.

Miller, W. R., & Rollnick, S. (2013). *Motivational interviewing: Helping people change* (3rd ed.). Guilford Press.

Miller, W. R., & Rollnick, S. (2023). *Motivational interviewing: Helping people change and grow.* Guildford Press.

Ponsford, J., Lee, N., Wong, D., McKay, A., Haines, K., Alway, Y., Downing, M., Furtado, C., & O'Donnell, M. (2015). Efficacy of motivational interviewing and cognitive behavioral therapy for anxiety and depression symptoms following traumatic brain injury. *Psychological Medicine, 46*(5), 1079–1090.

Poynter, L., Kwan, J., Sayer, A. A., & Vassallo, M. (2011). Does cognitive impairment affect rehabilitation outcome? *Journal of the American Geriatric Society, 59*(11), 2108–2111.

Prigatano, G. P. (2005). Therapy for emotional and motivational disorders. In W. M. High, Jr., A. M. Sander, M. A. Struchen, & K. A. Hart (Eds.), *Rehabilitation for traumatic brain injury* (pp. 118–130). Oxford University Press.

Randall, C. L., & McNeil, D. W. (2017). Motivational interviewing as an adjunct to cognitive behavior therapy for anxiety disorders: A critical review of the literature. *Cognitive and Behavioral Practice, 24*(3), 296–311.

Sendroy-Terrill, M., Whiteneck, G. G., & Brooks, C. A. (2010). Aging with traumatic brain injury: Cross-sectional follow-up of people receiving inpatient rehabilitation over more than three decades. *Archives of Physical Medicine and Rehabilitation, 91*(3), 489–497.

Sherer, M., Evans, C. C., Leverenz, J., Stouter, J., Irby, J. W., Jr., Lee, J. E., & Yablon, S. A. (2007). Therapeutic alliance in post-acute brain injury rehabilitation: Predictors of strength of alliance and impact of alliance on outcome. *Brain Injury, 21*(7), 663–672.

Worthington, A., & Wood, R. (2018). Apathy following traumatic brain injury: A review. *Neuropsychologia, 118*, 40–47.

Whyte, E., Skidmore, E., Aizenstein, H., Ricker, J., & Butters, M. (2011). Cognitive impairment in acquired brain injury: A predictor of rehabilitation outcomes and an opportunity for novel interventions. *Physical Medicine and Rehabilitation, 3*(6, S1), S45–S51.

Ylvisaker, M., Szekeres, S. F., & Feeney, T. J. (1998). Cognitive rehabilitation: Executive functions. In M. Ylvisaker (Ed.), *Traumatic brain injury rehabilitation: Children and adolescents* (pp. 221–269). Butterworth-Heinemann.

11 Family and Caregiver Dynamics
Asma Ali and Connie Jacocks

Description of Family and Caregiver Dynamics in Rehabilitation

In the United States, an estimated 53.0 million people provide informal care for another individual, with a prevalence equal to 1 in 5 (21.3%). This number has risen significantly over time due to the confluence of a number of factors including an aging population, limitations or workforce shortage in formal care systems, increased efforts by states to facilitate community and home-based services, and increased self-reporting of caregiving activities (AARP & National Alliance for Caregiving, 2020). Caregiving includes a range of activities such as providing assistance for basic and instrumental activities of daily living, emotional support, financial care, and mediation care.

There are many benefits to having a caregiver who is integrated into the care team, who is fully engaged and participatory in the inpatient and outpatient rehabilitation process, and who provides ongoing support through community reintegration. The quality of psychosocial and caregiver support is also known to have a direct impact on a range of outcomes in rehabilitation populations for both the caregiver and care recipient (Chwalisz & Dollinger, 2010). In addition, caregiver involvement can improve care recipients' access to services and reduce unmet needs. Integrating the

Asma Ali and Connie Jacocks, *Family and Caregiver Dynamics* In: *Motivational Interviewing in Medical Rehabilitation.*
Edited by: Nicole Schechter, Connie Jacocks, Lester Butt, and Stephen T. Wegener, Oxford University Press.
© Oxford University Press 2024. DOI: 10.1093/oso/9780197748268.003.0012

caregiver into care planning (including discharge) has been shown to reduce readmissions, shorten rehospitalizations, reduce post-discharge costs, and improve quality of life for the care recipient (Friedman & Tong, 2020; Rodakowski et al., 2017).

While there are many potential benefits, there are also significant challenges to caregiver participation in rehabilitation and the ability of caregivers to provide optimal support to their loved ones. For the caregiver, this might include the development of physical, psychological, or medical problems due to strain or burden associated with additional responsibilities. Unfortunately, the act of caregiving without appropriate supports can be associated with negative impacts to physical and mental health, including decreased well-being, depression, anxiety, health problems, social isolation, and financial loss, in addition to medical difficulties (e.g., reduced immune function, hypertension) and lead to disturbances in health behaviors such as sleep, alcohol use, and tobacco use (as reviewed in Chwalisz & Dollinger, 2010). Additional barriers to caregiver participation include caregivers' varying emotional readiness, physical ability, and confidence to engage in training. A care recipient's openness to assistance and desire for autonomy must also be balanced and may require navigation. Changing roles within the care dyad (e.g., an adult child taking care of their parent) can also introduce conflict.

This chapter explores such challenges in greater detail, within a solution-focused narrative. In particular, this chapter will discuss the use of motivational interviewing (MI) skills by rehabilitation professionals to navigate caregiver and care recipient dynamics within the rehabilitation setting. When working from a non-MI perspective, professionals tend to take on an expert role, provide authoritative directives, prematurely problem-solve, or pass judgment within interactions. This can contribute to a multitude of concerns including creating an imbalance within the relationship and fueling resistance or discord, thereby stunting the ability to create a collaborative relationship. In contrast, MI can be used to facilitate a collaborative partnership with the family/caregiver, to appreciate the potential ambivalence that may exist within an individual and between team members (e.g., values and beliefs of the family/caregiver in contrast to the care recipient, provider, or treatment team), to aid in the adjustment and preparedness of families/caregivers, as well as to encourage their participation in the care recipient's rehabilitation program.

Challenges in Family and Caregiver Dynamics

CAREGIVER ROLES AND RESPONSIBILITIES

Caregivers are considered key members on the rehabilitation team as they perform or assist with many roles that support care recipients' progression through rehabilitation. First, caregivers can play an essential role in providing assistance in self-cares. For example, many conditions such as spinal cord injury (SCI) and orthopedic injuries require many demands for self-management of disability, associated conditions (e.g., neurogenic bladder or bowel), and secondary complications (e.g., skin ulcers), directed by either the identified care recipient or a family/caregiver (Munce et al., 2014). The demands of caregiving also change as the care recipient's condition progresses or declines. Caregivers may be asked to learn new information quickly, adapt to the care recipient's changing needs, and assist and support in unfamiliar roles. In particular, discharge from a rehabilitation facility to home is a critical period of adjustment requiring significant learning and adaption for both the caregiver and care recipient (Ghazzawi et al., 2016).

Second, caregivers are often asked to assume the role of emotional support and to remain stalwart for the care recipient. In some cases, this responsibility can overshadow the care recipient's own emotional process as they too may be experiencing denial, grief, or loss. When a caregiver is themselves adjusting to the new condition while supporting the care recipient, their ability to learn and integrate information necessary to manage daily life moving forward may be negatively impacted (Rivera, 2012).

THE CARE DYAD

Given the bidirectional nature of the relationship between the caregiver and care recipient (also referred to as the *care dyad*), implications of caregiving and care receiving are important to consider for both parties. For example, high-quality caregiving can help prevent care recipients from experiencing secondary complications associated with SCI (Moreno et al., 2017; Munce et al., 2016). For caregivers, those who report greater ease with role adaptation during a care recipient's initial inpatient hospitalization are more likely to have better adjustment during those first 5 years post-injury or illness (Rivera, 2012). Additionally, within the stroke population, it has been shown that caregivers with positive coping and adequate social support are protected from negative implications associated with the caregiving role (Gibbs et al., 2020).

With regard to negative impacts, caregivers may experience physical, emotional, and financial strain, which can reduce the quality of care provided to the care recipient. Caregivers of individuals with SCI are more likely to experience physical distress and suffer from coronary heart disease and obesity, among other factors (Moreno et al., 2017). Within stroke populations it was found that caregiver depression worsened the depression of the care recipient, predicted poorer rehabilitation outcomes, and resulted in early discontinuation of home care (Grant et al., 2002). Further, it is important to note that the presence of cognitive impairment or communication disorders (affecting caregivers and/or care recipients) can complicate the care dyad. The reader may refer to Chapter 10 of this text for additional tools for the use of MI in these populations.

Preparing, integrating, and supporting caregivers themselves, as well as the care dyad, are thus vital. Jeyathevan et al. (2019) found that relationships between care recipients with SCI and caregivers can remain stable when the dyad applies skills such as interdependence, shifting commonalities, modifying routines, and creating a new normal.

BARRIERS TO CAREGIVER PARTICIPATION

Many challenges exist that can interfere in caregivers' ability or willingness to participate in care recipients' rehabilitation. After experiencing loss in emotional, physical, and functional facets of life, some care recipients look to maintain as much autonomy as possible, thereby declining caregivers' participation. While this may be concerning for the caregivers, there are benefits to the care recipient. When there is personal autonomy in independent functions, they are shown to experience personal and relational satisfaction, self-confidence, a sense of individual accomplishment in the completion of activities of daily living, and improved quality of life (Nikbakht-Nasrabadi et al., 2019).

Differences in values, or beliefs about disability and recovery, between the caregiver and care recipient can also present a barrier. Some examples of this include when the caregiver and care recipient do not align in their views on relationship dynamics, role definitions within the relationship, tasks that a partner or family member might/should perform within a medical setting, or when the care recipient should return to the community. Furthermore, caregivers and care recipients may hold different beliefs about disability identity and how the recovery course should or will look (Rivera, 2012).

When spouses and family members assume the caregiving role, the nature of the relationship often changes, causing asymmetrical dependency, loss of intimacy, and difficulty adapting (Jeyathevan et al., 2019). With such changes in roles, caregivers may experience loss of identity, social isolation and loneliness, and financial difficulties. For spouse caregiver and care recipient dyads in the first several years after an SCI, there is a higher incidence of separation and divorce due to challenges adapting to new physical functions (Kreuter et al., 1998). Further, parents giving care to children experience higher levels of stress than spousal caregivers. Tasks may become unevenly distributed among family members, leading to increased stress in communication, family unity, power structure, and interpersonal relationships (Jeyathevan et al., 2019). A longer duration of caregiving has also been associated with poorer quality of life (Lynch & Cahalan, 2017).

Importance of Intervention

Intervention to support caregivers, care recipients, and the care dyad improves the health of all parties. In fact, providing support to both parties is one of the strongest predictors of community participation (Erler et al., 2019; Grant et al., 2002). Grant et al. (2002) found that family caregivers who participated in a social problem-solving intervention group had better problem-solving skills; greater preparedness; less depression; significant improvement in measures of vitality, social functioning, and mental health; and fewer role limitations related to emotional problems. In addition, specific dyadic coping strategies such as focusing on the present, focusing on reasonable goals, and positive reframing were found to be beneficial when incorporated into cognitive and communication coping interventions (Robinson-Smith et al., 2016).

MI is another intervention that can be helpful to the care dyad. In general, MI is a unique and powerful tool for promoting participation in these activities aimed at reducing potential challenges the caregiver and care dyad may experience, while maximizing benefit and outcomes. Vellone et al. (2020) demonstrated that integration of MI skills into patient education improved self-care in individuals with heart failure, and this was potentiated by caregiver participation. A follow-up analysis of this same study group indicated reduced mortality in patients with heart failure if caregivers were included in the intervention (Iovino et al., 2021). There are many opportunities within rehabilitation contexts to integrate the spirit and principles of MI to promote caregiver engagement in rehabilitation and provide essential caregiver support. The tools of MI can be utilized to do the following:

- Establish rapport with caregivers and families
- Facilitate a collaborative working relationship with caregivers
- Provide education to caregivers that is approachable and well received
- Explore personal values and beliefs of caregivers
- Explore discord among the care dyad
- Support dialogue between the care dyad and treatment team
- Facilitate transitions from care facilities to the home
- Monitor emotional adjustment of caregivers

MI-SPECIFIC SKILLS FOR NAVIGATING FAMILY AND CAREGIVER DYNAMICS

Unique circumstances often surround family/caregiver involvement within the rehabilitation setting. As mentioned earlier, some families/caregivers readily assume the caregiving role (e.g., obligation, commitment, submitting to internal/external pressures or factors). However, others may experience challenges or display reluctance toward participation. In these circumstances a provider can use basic and/or advanced MI skills to foster development of collaborative dialogue.

Basic attitudes such as partnership, acceptance, collaboration/compassion, and empowerment/empathy create a foundation upon which trust and safety can be built. For example, if caregivers are reluctant or ambivalent to participate in cares, the provider can demonstrate partnership by eliciting caregiver beliefs: "Tell me what your thoughts are on your role in relation to the care recipient." Additional MI skills, such as open-ended questions, affirmations, reflections, and summaries (OARS), can be used to facilitate collaborative interactions. For instance, it is common that caregivers hold different beliefs from someone on the care team (care recipient's, providers, or treatment team's perspective or beliefs). To further rather than stunt discourse, it could be helpful to use reflections and open-ended questions: "You seem to have a different opinion than the physician and team on how recovery will look." (Reflection). "Tell me more about this?" (Open-ended question). The reader may also refer to Chapter 3 to review the foundational MI skills.

Various advanced skills can be used by team members to promote collaboration between caregivers and the team or caregivers and the patient. A provider could use elaboration to evoke change talk and learn more when caregivers present with emotional, physical, and/or cognitive concerns that impede their ability to participate. For example, "What would be helpful to prevent you from feeling overloaded?" In another example in which caregiver responsibility may be unevenly distributed among family members, querying extremes can also be used to evoke change talk: "What are some good things that might happen if you decided to involve other family members in training?"

Advanced skills can also be applied when working with a caregiver who is using sustain talk. For example, a caregiver may be refusing to turn a care recipient with SCI during the night to provide pressure relief. This caregiver may verbalize, "We're prioritizing getting sleep together, and there have been no skin issues." A provider could follow up by using a skill such as *agreeing with a twist*: "You're accustomed to sleeping through the night together. I can see how that would be a priority for you." In another example, a caregiver may possess certain beliefs about what it means to be a supportive partner and may say "I can't take a day off. He needs me here, and it's important to me to be the best partner, even if I burn out." A *running head start* can be applied here by responding, "Tell me more about what you have enjoyed about being here every day. What would be beneficial if you were to take a day off for yourself?"

In general, infusing the working relationship with MI spirit is key when working with caregivers and families and in supporting the caregiver dyad. A combination of MI spirit (PACE), foundational MI skills (OARS), as well as more advanced skills can be used to facilitate collaborative interactions. Readers are encouraged to relate PACE, OARS, and advanced skills outlined in Tables 11.1–11.3, respectively, to the transcripts that follow.

TABLE 11.1

Motivational Interviewing Spirit (PACE) Applied to Families/Caregivers

Partnership	Definition: Providers and families/caregivers align to work together collaboratively, in a nonhierarchical dynamic.
	Application: The provider invites family/caregiver to share their ideas prior to sharing their own ideas.
	Example: "What would help you to feel like a part of the team?"
Acceptance	Definition: Families/caregivers have the right to make decisions that may be contrary to what a provider thinks and feels regarding the family/caregiver circumstance(s).
	Application: The provider respects the contrasting decision made by a family/caregiver regarding discharge plans, which is not consistent with clinical recommendations.
	Example: "We worry about the safety of the home environment yet understand that you are working to the best of your ability to make it safe given the resources available."
Compassion	Definition: Providers foster developing a united relationship with families/caregivers.
	Application: The provider works jointly with the family/caregiver in listening and learning what their values are.
	Example: "Tell me more about what you are specifically hoping to learn in the final few weeks here."
Empowerment	Definition: The belief that the family/caregiver and patient have within them what they need to make change is fundamental within provider–family/caregiver dynamics. This creates opportunity to ask questions surrounding behavioral change and explore all perspectives.
	Application: As a trusting relationship is established between the provider and family/caregiver, the provider is able to ask permission about offering professional knowledge and information.
	Example: "Would it be OK with you if I talk through the steps of the bowel program?"

TABLE 11.2

Motivational Interviewing Foundational Skills (OARS) Applied to Families/Caregivers

Open-ended question	Example: "What don't I know about your relationship and connectedness with the care recipient that would be helpful for me to understand?"
Affirmation	Example: "You've got a compassionate heart and care so deeply for the care recipient."
Reflection	Example: "You're confident in handling their care already."
Summary	Example: "Let me see if I have this right. You've been there from the start, supporting and caring for the care recipient while in the intensive care unit. You're a strong advocate for the care recipient and strive to ensure that safety and quality care are being delivered. You've absorbed so much information about cares already and feel confident in your current caretaking skills, and you're eager to learn all you can prior to going home. Would it be OK if I share some information about how we train here and what might be different than what you've previously learned at the intensive care unit?"

Case Study

PART 1: CARE RECIPIENT AND PSYCHOLOGIST

The care recipient is an adult male who sustained an acute traumatic cervical SCI. The care recipient's wife is participating in his rehabilitation program to learn and assist with cares. The care recipient is open and receptive and welcomes family training; however, his wife is apprehensive about learning and participating in cares. Read below to see how MI is infused in this conversation.

PSYCHOLOGIST: "Hi there, how is it going today?"

CARE RECIPIENT: "Doc, it is not going well at all."

PSYCHOLOGIST: "It sounds like you are feeling upset about something." (Emotion reflection)

CARE RECIPIENT: "Yeah, I am really concerned about my wife. She is not doing well with all this. The injury, my needs, my cares . . . they are all too much for her."

PSYCHOLOGIST: "Tell me a little more about your concerns?" (Open-ended question)

CARE RECIPIENT: "See here, I am ready for my wife to start learning my cares. We only have a few weeks left until discharge, and there is a lot for her to learn. I want her to know how to do things, but I do not think she is ready. I do not think she wants to."

TABLE 11.3

Motivational Interviewing Advanced Skills Applied to Families/Caregivers

Advanced skill for listening for change talk

Preparatory talk—need	Definition: A precommitment for change talk that occurs in which a necessity is verbalized in dialogue for a change to occur (Rollnick et al., 2008). Example: Family/caregiver states, "I need to get some more sleep."

Advanced skills for building motivation for change

Evocative question	Definition: Using open-ended questions in a direct fashion when exploring ambivalence and specific concerns that exist (Miller & Rollnick, 2002). Example: The provider says to a family/caregiver, "What would you be willing to try?"
Elaboration	Definition: Having a family/caregiver provide additional details on a topic prior to moving to another topic, specifically when a reason for change has been vocalized (Miller & Rollnick, 2002). Example: Provider says to the family/caregiver, "In what ways would it be helpful to learn more about skin safety?"

Advanced skills for responding to sustain talk and discord

Amplified reflection	Definition: Reflecting what the family/caregiver has said, with amplification or exaggeration. This can trigger the care recipient to step back and elicit the other side of ambivalence (Miller & Rollnick, 2002). Example: Provider's response to a family/caregiver who feels like they do not need any more bowel training, "It seems to you that you have learned the process very well, with no need for additional practice."
Double-sided reflection	Definition: Reflecting the resistant side of the argument and the ambivalent side based on arguments previously voiced by the family/caregiver. It is important to use conjunctions such as *and* and *yet* to maintain a balance, while starting with the sustain talk and ending on the change talk statement (Miller & Rollnick, 2002). Example: Provider says to the family/caregiver, "On the one hand, you are so busy and it is simpler to keep canceling your own psychotherapy appointments, yet, on the other hand, you are feeling overwhelmed with all the changes and want some support."

(*continued*)

TABLE 11.3 *Continued*

Emphasizing autonomy	Definition: Providing early assurances that a family/caregiver ultimately decides outcomes for themselves. This is a skill that is best used when resistance, or sustain talk and discord, occurs in which a family/caregiver perceives their freedom of making choices is being threatened. Therefore, the individual chooses to assert their preference (Miller & Rollnick, 2002; Miller & Rollnick, 2023).
	Example: The provider says to the family/caregiver, "This is just information on home modifications to assist with bathroom accessibility. What you decide to do is completely up to you; no one can make you build those plans."
Coming alongside	Definition: Using collaborative dialogue to help the family/caregiver explore ambivalence, specifically both sides of the argument. Siding with the counterchange perspective of the argument should help in eliciting change talk from the family/caregiver (Miller & Rollnick, 2002).
	Example: The provider says to the family/caregiver, "It may just be worth it to you to sell your house and move closer to the hospital, despite all the logistical stressors, so your spouse can continue rehab. It's worth the cost."

PSYCHOLOGIST: "You are feeling the time crunch approaching and worry about her openness." (Emotion reflection)

CARE RECIPIENT: "Well yeah, I am. I keep asking her to learn and telling her there is a checklist, but she keeps telling me we have time, and she will get to it. I want to give her time, I have been giving her time, but she is not ready. It's as if she is afraid. It's as if she doesn't want to learn."

PSYCHOLOGIST: "You're considerate and care a lot about the well-being and coping of your wife, and you want to respect her needs." (Affirmation)

CARE RECIPIENT: "Yeah. If it were me in her shoes, I would have learned everything already. She is very different from me though. I just do not know what else to do."

PSYCHOLOGIST: "You are feeling really stuck right now. It sounds like you have had many hard conversations with her about your concerns, and it feels as if it is not going anywhere." (Reflection)

CARE RECIPIENT: "Pretty much."

PSYCHOLOGIST: "What do you think might be helpful for your wife?" (Open-ended question)

CARE RECIPIENT: "I think she needs help adjusting to all this as much as I do. And maybe some help in prioritizing what is most important. She seems so overwhelmed, and I'm worried we won't get to the most important things."

PSYCHOLOGIST: "You want her to have some help in all of this, to feel less stressed and more focused." (Reflection)

CARE RECIPIENT: "Yes, exactly."

PSYCHOLOGIST: "Would it be OK if I check in with your wife to talk more about this?" (Asking permission)

CARE RECIPIENT: "Yeah, that would be great. Thanks Doc."

The spirit of MI was instrumental in this case. The psychologist and care recipient had a very collaborative dynamic. They had been working together several times per week, and through the course of treatment, the care recipient became increasingly comfortable with talking about concerns and emotions related to their injury and adjustment. Furthermore, emotional reflections offered by the psychologist helped in fostering a sense of safety with processing his thoughts and feelings. Establishment of this rapport allowed the psychologist to use MI foundational skills when needed. This allowed the psychologist to learn more about what was distressing the care recipient. A reflection of emotion was used to elicit details about how the care recipient was feeling. He readily began expressing concerns, which allowed the psychologist to use open-ended questions to gather additional details while deepening empathy within the relational dynamic. Simple content reflections were interspersed throughout the dialogue, reaffirming that the provider was accurately listening. An affirmation was also used to highlight the care recipient's character and values related to their relationship with their spouse. Lastly, an opportunity arose for the psychologist to ask permission to meet with the family/caregiver, to explore barriers to training from their perspective.

PART 2: CAREGIVER (WIFE) AND PSYCHOLOGIST

PSYCHOLOGIST: "Hello, how are you doing today?"

WIFE: "I do not even know where to start."

PSYCHOLOGIST: "You have a lot on your mind." (Reflection)

WIFE: "Yeah, there is just so much I am thinking about."

PSYCHOLOGIST: "You are overwhelmed with it all." (Emotion reflection)

WIFE: "I am. This has been so hard. There is so much to do. I am trying to take care of so much right now. I am spending my days here, still working, and trying to plan for all the changes that need to happen when we go home."

PSYCHOLOGIST: "You are juggling a lot right now." (Reflection)

WIFE: "I am, but I feel like I am not doing enough. I feel like I am failing at it all."

PSYCHOLOGIST: "Tell me a little bit more about why you feel like you are failing at it all?" (Open-ended question)

WIFE: "Well, for one, my husband wants me here all the time. But I cannot be. I need time to take care of things. I need time for work or planning for things we need when we return home. He wants me here all the time and keeps telling me I need to learn his cares. I have got so much other stuff going on that needs to be taken care of, and he does not understand that those are priorities too. There is not enough time to do everything, and I am failing at it all. I am letting everyone down. I am letting him down. I cannot seem to do anything right."

PSYCHOLOGIST: "It sounds like you are feeling pulled in many directions and that there is not enough time to do what you want or need. You are a hard worker and accustomed to planning and getting things done. Right now, there is just too much on your plate, and when you feel like you cannot get to it all, it leaves you feeling negatively about yourself." (Summary)

WIFE: "Yeah, that is the case. You know, I did not ask for this. I am scared out of my mind."

PSYCHOLOGIST: "You feel scared about all these changes." (Emotion reflection)

WIFE: "I sure am. I love my husband so much, but I feel like I don't know how to be here for him. I cannot know what he is going through. This has to be hard for him, but it is also hard for me. I feel like I cannot tell him how hard it is for me, because this is happening to him. He is the one who is injured. When I share how I feel overwhelmed he gets so upset and emotional. I feel like I am not allowed to have negative emotions because of what he is going through."

PSYCHOLOGIST: "You are a loving and supportive wife, and you want to be here for your husband, even if that means putting your emotions to the side." (Affirmation, amplified reflection)

WIFE: "It is as if he does not want to hear what is going on with me and what I need."

PSYCHOLOGIST: "You are overwhelmed and sometimes feel unheard. At the same time, you want to continue being his support, no matter what the cost." (Coming alongside)

WIFE: "I do want to keep helping him, but I feel like I am letting him down all the time. I just need some time to get other things wrapped up. I do not need him coming at me or telling me more things 'I have to do.'" (Preparatory talk—need)

PSYCHOLOGIST: "It is really up to you to decide if and when you feel ready to take on more." (Emphasizing autonomy)

WIFE: "It is. I know I will get there, but I just want to get there when I am ready, not when my husband tells me I need to be ready."

PSYCHOLOGIST: "On the one hand, you do not feel ready to take this on—the cares, the responsibilities. On the other hand, you know you will be able to do it when you have taken care of and crossed some other things off your list." (Double-sided reflection)

WIFE: "Yeah, that is true. I love my husband, and I will do what I need to, in order to help him. I just need him to stop pressuring me and making me feel bad for not being here all the time and working on his timeline. There is so much other stuff that has to get done."

PSYCHOLOGIST: "Tell me how you might know when you have gotten some things cleared off your plate?" (Open-ended question)

WIFE: "Well, for one, it will be when I have knocked some of this stuff off my list. I have a few work deadlines to meet, and I have to check out some vehicles. We are going to need a new car for us to be able to get around in the future, and I have some great options to check out while here. After those are checked off, I will feel like there is more time to be here and present."

PSYCHOLOGIST: "It sounds like you want to carve out some time to do what you need, and then you will feel ready to be here with your husband." (Reflection)

WIFE: "Yeah, that would make it so much easier."

PSYCHOLOGIST: "How might you go about scheduling some of this time you need?" (Evocative question)

WIFE: "Well, I guess I should talk to my husband and just let him know I need some blocks of time to get things done. We can look at his schedule and see what might work for that this week. Then I can plan to be here more regularly, and I will be ready to learn his cares."

PSYCHOLOGIST: "It sounds like you are feeling confident and have plans to take care of some business." (Reflection)

WIFE: "Yeah, I do. I think this helped a lot. I feel like I know how to manage this all better for my husband and myself."

In this conversation, the psychologist used the MI spirit to build a working and collaborative relationship and to explore the caregiver's thoughts and feelings related to her adjustment process, stressors, and personal ambivalence. The psychologist promoted exploration of the caregiver's ambivalence by navigating sustain talk in a way that was normalizing and supportive. This, in turn, encouraged a shift in ambivalence toward behavior change. Once change talk was established, the psychologist used open-ended questions, reflections, and an evocative question to elicit deeper exploration of the caregiver's ideas for successfully engaging in her husband's rehabilitation plan.

In sum, the psychologist was able to use these principles and skills to help the caregiver explore both sides of her ambivalence regarding engagement in family training and strategically guide the caregiver toward behavior change.

Summary

Integrating the caregiver into rehabilitation remains a vital component of comprehensive interdisciplinary care. Caregivers are essential to the rehabilitation and community success of individuals with illness and injury, and there are many opportunities to integrate the spirit and principles of MI in working with the care dyad. MI can be utilized in this context to facilitate a collaborative working relationship, provide education, explore personal values and beliefs, navigate discord within the care dyad, promote dialogue between the care dyad and treatment team, and monitor emotional adjustment. In general, the use of MI can create opportunity for improved engagement and benefit for all individuals participating in the rehabilitation program.

References

AARP & National Alliance for Caregiving. (2020). *Caregiving in the United States 2020.*

Chwalisz, K., & Dollinger, S. C. (2010). Evidence-based practice with family caregivers: Decision-making strategies based on research and clinical data. In R. G. Frank, M. Rosenthal, & B. Caplan (Eds.), *Handbook of rehabilitation psychology* (2nd ed., pp. 301–311). American Psychological Association.

Erler, K. S., Sullivan, V., Mckinnon, S., & Inzana, R. (2019). Social support as a predictor of community participation after stroke. *Frontiers in Neurology, 10,* Article 1013.

Friedman, E. M., & Tong, P. K. (2020). *A framework for integrating family caregivers into the health care team.* RAND Corporation.

Ghazzawi, A., Kuziemsky, C., & O'Sullivan, T. (2016). Using a complex adaptive system lens to understand family caregiving experiences navigating the stroke rehabilitation system. *BMC Health Services Research, 16*(1), Article 538.

Gibbs, L. A. L., Anderson, M. I., Simpson, G. K., & Jones, K. F. (2020). Spirituality and resilience among family caregivers of survivors: A scoping review. *NeuroRehabilitation, 46*(1), 41–52.

Grant, J. S., Elliott, T. R., Weaver, M., Bartolucci, A. A., & Giger, J. N. (2002). Telephone intervention with family caregivers of stroke survivors after rehabilitation. *Stroke, 33*(8), 2060–2065.

Iovino, P., Rebora, P., Occhino, G., Zeffiro, V., Caggianelli, G., Ausili, D., Alvaro, R., Riegel, B., & Vellone, E. (2021). Effectiveness of motivational interviewing on health-service use and mortality: A secondary outcome analysis of the MOTIVATE-HF trial. *ESC Heart Failure, 8*(4), 2920–2927.

Jeyathevan, G., Cameron, J. I., Craven, B. C., Munce, S. E. P., & Jaglal, S. B. (2019). Re-building relationships after a spinal cord injury: Experiences of family caregivers and care recipients. *BMC Neurology, 19,* Article 117.

Kreuter, M., Sullivan, M., Dahllöf, A. G., & Siösteen, A. (1998). Partner relationships, functioning, mood and global quality of life in persons with spinal cord injury and traumatic brain injury. *Spinal Cord, 36*(4), 252–261.

Lynch, J., & Cahalan, R. (2017). The impact of spinal cord injury on the quality of life of primary family caregivers: A literature review. *Spinal Cord, 55*(11), 964–978.

Miller, W. R., & Rollnick, S. (2002). *Motivational interviewing: Preparing people for change* (2nd ed.). Guilford Press.

Miller, W.R., & Rollnick, S. (2023). *Motivational interviewing: Helping people change and grow.* Guilford Press.

Moreno, A., Zidarov, D., Raju, C., Boruff, J., & Ahmed, S. (2017). Integrating the perspectives of individuals with spinal cord injuries, their family caregivers and healthcare professionals from the time of rehabilitation admission to community reintegration: Protocol for a scoping study on SCI needs. *BMJ Open, 7*(8), Article e014331.

Munce, S. E., Webster, F., Fehlings, M. G., Straus, S. E., Jang, E., & Jaglal, S. B. (2014). Perceived facilitators and barriers to self-management in individuals with traumatic spinal cord injury: A qualitative descriptive study. *BMC Neurology, 14*, Article 48.

Nikbakht-Nasrabadi, A., Mohammadi, N., Yazdanshenas, M., & Shabany, M. (2019). Toward overcoming physical disability in spinal cord injury: A qualitative inquiry of the experiences of injured individuals and their families. *BMC Neurology, 19*, Article 171.

Rivera, P. A. (2012). Families in rehabilitation. In P. Kennedy (Ed.), *The Oxford handbook of rehabilitation psychology* (pp. 160–170). Oxford University Press.

Robinson-Smith, G., Harmer, C., Sheeran, R., & Bellino Vallo, E. (2016). Couples' coping after stroke—A pilot intervention study. *Rehabilitation Nursing, 41*(4), 218–229.

Rodakowski, J., Rocco, P. B., Ortiz, M., Folb, B., Schulz, R., Morton, S. C., Leathers, S. C., Hu, L., & James, A. E., 3rd. (2017). Caregiver integration during discharge planning for older adults to reduce resource use: A meta-analysis. *Journal of the American Geriatrics Society, 65*(8), 1748–1755.

Rollnick, S., Miller, W. R., & Butler, C. C. (2008). *Motivational interviewing in health care: Helping care recipients change behavior.* Guilford Press.

Vellone, E., Rebora, P., Ausili, D., Zeffiro, V., Pucciarelli, G., Caggianelli, Masci, S., Alvaro, R., & Riegel, B. (2020) Motivational interviewing to improve self-care in heart failure patients (MOTIVATE-HF): A randomized controlled trial. *ESC Heart Failure, 7*, 1309–1318.

SECTION III

Implementation and Evaluation

12 Motivational Interviewing Training, Training Resources, and System Change

Nicole Schechter and Laura Torres

Introduction

As the earlier portions of this book have described, motivational interviewing (MI) is an invaluable approach for use with patients, families, and interdisciplinary team members in the rehabilitation setting. Unfortunately, few rehabilitation clinicians receive formal training in MI during their professional education. Therefore, individual clinicians, practice management, and/or hospital/organizational leadership may identify MI as an important training target.

MI Training Approaches

Rehabilitation professionals, practices, and institutions may consider a range of factors when determining the MI training process, including who to train and when to train. Some simply encourage individual rehabilitation professionals to seek out their own MI training, some opt to train small groups of professionals, while others take a system-level approach. No approach fits all, and there is no "right" or "wrong" way to pursue MI training.

Nicole Schechter and Laura Torres, *Motivational Interviewing Training, Training Resources, and System Change* In: *Motivational Interviewing in Medical Rehabilitation*. Edited by: Nicole Schechter, Connie Jacocks, Lester Butt, and Stephen T. Wegener, Oxford University Press. © Oxford University Press 2024. DOI: 10.1093/oso/9780197748268.003.0013

WHO TO TRAIN

In some instances, allowing individual rehabilitation professionals to independently pursue their own MI training is appropriate. In this approach, depending on the organization's resources and policies, individual professionals may receive reimbursement for training costs or dedicated time away from work to pursue their own professional development. Since in this approach professionals are self-selecting into training, it ensures that they believe MI training is important and applicable to their work. According to adult learning theory (Knowles, 1984), they are therefore more likely to integrate MI into their clinical practice.

In other instances, an organization may identify a specific workflow problem or patient satisfaction challenge that could be improved or addressed with the integration of effective MI. As such, the organization might dedicate time and resources toward MI training for a small group of professionals involved in that particular segment of care. As an example, an organization may identify that patients are completing their brief telephonic intake session but not following through on their in-person initial therapy evaluation. Consequently, the organization may wish to provide MI training for the professionals conducting the telephonic intakes. In this quality improvement approach, the organization must be thoughtful about how it introduces the purpose of the training, how and why the trainees have been selected, and how the effects of the training will be measured. Risks of this approach include that professionals feel singled out for poor performance or believe that the training is punitive. Please review Chapter 13 for more information about this approach.

Another approach may be to expose an entire workforce to MI training. The training itself may take many forms; however, applying a system-wide approach requires many considerations. First, organizational leadership must understand and be able to explain the evidence base for MI and how MI training connects to the organizational mission and willing to commit staff time and therefore monetary resources to the training. It is most helpful when leaders identify targets that MI can address and are willing to devote resources to measure outcomes. Second, organizational leadership must commit to a long-term initiative; MI training cannot be a "flavor of the week." This is best demonstrated when MI training or growth in MI skills becomes integrated into clinical staff performance reviews over a period and when staff are even incentivized to demonstrate growth in MI skills. Similarly, organizational leaders must participate in the MI training efforts and might consider integrating MI into managerial or supervision processes. As an example, when a manager attends an MI workshop with their team and subsequently uses MI in a staff meeting, the team is more likely to use MI in turn. Third, it will be important for rehabilitation team leaders, often physicians, to demonstrate buy-in by attending training with their fellow team members and utilizing MI in patient care and team interactions. Please refer to Chapter 6 for more information on how MI can be used in the context of rehabilitation teams.

Supporting an entire system of clinicians to become competent in MI can be quite challenging as this takes considerable time and resources. To be considered competent in MI, individuals must be able to demonstrate adequate and consistent MI knowledge, MI spirit, and MI skills. To accomplish this requires significant self-study or training in workshops, plus many opportunities for practicing MI skills with evaluation and feedback from those already deemed to be competent in high-quality MI. One common system-level approach to training is to identify members in the organization who are already competent in MI and can serve as trainers or identify those who might be interested in becoming competent in MI to serve as trainers. Then, these trainers provide introductory MI workshops for the workforce so that a substantial portion of the staff are exposed to foundational MI concepts and skills; this helps the workforce "speak the same language" with patients and one another. Through participation in these workshops, individuals who are particularly enthusiastic or interested in MI can volunteer to serve as on-site MI champions.

Once on-site champions are identified, the organization can dedicate extra time and resources to more intensive training for these professionals. These champions, along with on-site MI trainers, become responsible for providing the rest of the workforce with opportunities for developing and integrating MI skills into daily practice. It is recommended that these opportunities be focused on MI skills that are specific to the clinical setting rather than expecting that the entire workforce become competent in the general foundational principles, tasks, and skills of MI. For example, champions and on-site trainers may lead a monthly or quarterly case discussion in which the team discusses what and how MI may be used to guide the patient forward. Those leading the case discussion can use MI themselves to model the skills.

WHEN TO TRAIN

Determining the appropriate time for MI training in part depends on who is being trained. Generally speaking, there is not a "wrong" time for an individual rehabilitation professional to pursue MI training. However, consistent with MI principles, the individual will benefit from participating in training when they believe it is important to them (i.e., applicable to their work, beneficial in some way, abetting their patient relationships, and augmenting quality outcomes and collaboration) and when they are confident they can devote the necessary time, energy, and attention to the training.

The same concept applies to organizations making training available (or mandatory) to staff at a small group level or system-wide. It is imperative that organizations implement MI training when such an initiative can be prioritized from the top down and from the bottom up, which may include tying the value of MI training to other organizational focuses. For example, if an organization recently began an initiative to improve the levels of activity and mobility for hospitalized patients, MI training can be very useful in helping staff minimize patient refusals or motivate patients for hospital activity. In other circumstances, it may be that a previously identified hospital initiative is too taxing, so MI training should be delayed.

Just like individual readiness can be measured using MI techniques that have been discussed earlier in this book, organizational readiness for engagement in MI training can and should be measured prior to MI training implementation. There are several standardized measures of organizational readiness that may be used, including, but not limited to, the Organizational Readiness for Implementing Change (Shea et al., 2014) and the Organizational Readiness to Change Assessment (Helfrich et al., 2009).

For some groups, the answer to "when to train" comes down entirely to minimizing financial burden as the greatest costs of MI training are often those incurred when closing clinics, taking staff off rotations, or asking staff to engage in training during already scheduled time off. Thus, it can be useful to embed training into new staff orientation. In addition to minimizing financial burden, this demonstrates the organization's prioritization of MI as part of staff and patient care culture. Other methods for minimizing financial burden on the institution include completion of MI training after clinical hours are complete or during staff lunch breaks. These options require dividing training into small chunks (i.e., 1-hour or 2-hour training sessions) that are repeated weekly or monthly. When asking clinicians to participate in training outside of regular business hours, offering incentives is recommended.

HOW TO TRAIN

Preexisting staff MI knowledge will vary based on their clinical experience and previous training experiences and should be taken into consideration when developing a training program. A needs and knowledge assessment completed in advance will help the training target knowledge gaps, which will make it especially useful and relevant to the staff. No matter what gaps in knowledge are identified, all MI training should be rooted in key principles of adult learning theory, including andragogy (Knowles, 1984) and transformative learning (Mezirow, 1991). *Andragogy* is a teaching method where "real-world problems" are incorporated and learners are given the opportunity to self-direct their learning in some ways. For example, an andragogy-consistent training for occupational therapists (OTs) would involve role-playing MI skills during an activities of daily living treatment session and inviting the OTs to select if they would like to watch a video demonstration, a live role-play of skills, or play an MI skill development game. Transformative learning theory conceptualizes that adults learn best when engaged in a process of reflection. This can be accomplished in many ways, but one example involves learners role-playing a specific scenario and then debriefing in a small group what went well during the role-play and what they would like to try differently next time.

These principles point to the importance of forgoing lecturing or exclusively didactic methods for experiential learning with opportunities for customization and skills practice. The Motivational Interviewing Network of Trainers (MINT) outlines on its website some guidelines and recommended approaches for introductory, intermediate, and advanced MI trainings (https://motivationalinterviewing. org/training-expectations).

TRAINING MODELS

MI training can be accomplished in many different formats and combinations, including asynchronous e-learning programs, virtual workshops, and in-person workshops. Please see Table 12.1 for a summary of these options. When selecting the format(s) for training, it is perhaps most important to ensure that it is accessible and feasible for the audience. Putting an MI e-learning course on the organization's learning management system, which already houses electronic courses for compliance with policies and best practices, increases access and allows the organization to track who completes the course and with what level of competence. Another example is conducting a live MI workshop during an already scheduled 1-hour team meeting for a few consecutive weeks. Asking rehabilitation teams to add meetings to their already busy schedules decreases accessibility and decreases the level of staff engagement once they arrive to the training.

Advantages to e-learning programs include the ability for learners to access the material from anywhere at any time and to self-pace the training. That is, a learner can stop and start the training as many times as needed given the learner's schedule and other responsibilities. Disadvantages of e-learning programs include the inability to customize to a specific learner's work setting or discipline, lack of opportunity to practice MI skills and receive immediate feedback, and costs associated with purchasing or creating such a program. As mentioned earlier, e-learning programs can be hosted on an organization's existing learning management system, or an organization may opt to use an external e-learning platform, like Second Life, that can be easily accessed via weblinks or at kiosks.

TABLE 12.1

Motivational Interviewing Training Methods

Training method	Description	Advantages	Disadvantages
Self-study	Identifying resources that one can consume (i.e., books, journal articles, podcasts) to increase competence	• Self-paced • Self-direct to most interesting and relevant material/customization • Convenience/accessibility	• Minimal accountability • Minimal opportunity for practicing skills • Minimal opportunity for exchange of ideas • Uncertainty about which resources to select
E-learning	Training via an asynchronous program available online	• Self-paced • Convenience/accessibility • Important information preselected • Potential for CE/CME	• Minimal self-direction/customization • Minimal opportunity for practicing skills • Minimal opportunity for exchange of ideas • Cost
Live workshops	Training that involves exchange of ideas and skills practice that is led by a field expert	• Important information preselected • Potential for CE/CME • Opportunity for practicing skills	• Reduced convenience/accessibility • Minimal self-direction/customization • Cost
Combination	Training that combines two or three of the above options	• Can allow for more advanced skill development • Optimizes advantages and minimizes disadvantages of the individual training options	• Requires more time and effort

Note: CE = continuing education; CME = continuing medical education.

Considerations when purchasing or creating an e-learning MI training program are ensuring that the program functions on both computers and smartphones, includes foundational MI content, engages adult learners using a variety of modalities, and is accessible for individuals with a range of disabilities (Thomson et al., 2015). Additionally, it is important that the creators of the program are considered MI experts, with at least one being a MINT member, and that the development team sought feedback from key stakeholders, including patients and families.

Live workshop training can be conducted in person or virtually and can range in length. One advantage of live workshops, in-person or virtual, is the ability to customize the training experience to match the level of knowledge and the discipline or work setting of the audience. Another advantage is the opportunity for exchange between the trainer and audience and between audience members. Live workshops also give opportunities for trainers, MI experts, to demonstrate skills and for learners to practice skills. This is less easily accomplished in virtual workshops because though learners can be sent into virtual breakout rooms to practice skills, this requires that all learners are in private spaces connected via their own electronic device. Additionally, it can be challenging for trainers to get to all virtual breakout rooms to provide ample feedback. Disadvantages of live workshop training, in-person or virtual, are complications of scheduling and costs associated with closing clinics or taking professionals off units to participate. If an organization does not have internal trainers, it would have to hire an MI trainer.

These diverse types of training can be combined to meet the many needs of the learners. Learners often respond well to hybrid training that combines both asynchronous and synchronous learning opportunities. A combination creates more flexibility for the learner, allowing them to complete a portion of training at their own pace during times that are most convenient for them and still providing opportunities in live workshops to practice skills and receive feedback, observe, and ask questions.

HOW ARE MI SKILLS MAINTAINED?

Although research has shown that live workshops usually produce some immediate improvements in MI knowledge and skills, these gains can be quickly lost (Soderlund et al., 2011). Miller and Mount (2001) showed that MI skill level decreased after approximately 4 months if skills are not being regularly practiced and if individuals are not receiving personal performance feedback. Therefore, it is useful to identify practical methods in which individuals or groups of learners can engage to support maintenance of skills after initial training.

Participation in regular MI coaching and feedback sessions can play an important role in sustainability of skills (Schwalbe et al., 2014). Such sessions might involve reviewing recorded patient–provider conversations or treatment sessions so that individual learners are held accountable to practice MI skills between sessions and evolve skills after receiving feedback from MI trainers. Another, less time-intensive option is to incorporate a brief MI discussion or MI skills practice activity into a monthly staff meeting. These activities can vary in length and can take as little as 10–15 minutes. The activities can be led by the learners on a rotating basis or by a volunteer MI "champion" supported by organizational leaders to grow and enhance MI knowledge and skills in the organization.

MI Training Content

Training content may vary depending on the knowledge, skill level, goals, and availability of the learning group. Assuming that most rehabilitation learner groups have limited prior MI knowledge, training content should at minimum include an overview of MI, a review of ambivalence and readiness for change, change and sustain talk, MI spirit (acceptance, compassion, empowerment;), and the basic MI skills (open-ended questions, affirmations, reflections, summaries; Soderlund et al., 2011). Introductory trainings that last a portion of a day up to a full day will focus on exposing learners to the aforementioned topics and helping them determine if they want to learn more about MI and how to continue developing MI skills through their own practice.

Introductory training sessions that are several days long, with spacing in between (i.e., 2 weeks between sessions) are more likely to support skill development. Intermediate and advanced levels of training are less commonly needed, especially when implementing MI training at a system level. If individual learners have established MI skills and would like to pursue intermediate and advanced MI training, these can be sought out via the MINT website (https://motivationalinterview ing.org/list-events). Another option is creating small groups within the organization for individuals who are interested in furthering their MI competencies. Small groups can hold consistent meetings during which self-study occurs and MI is discussed.

Prior to identifying an MI training curriculum or an MI trainer to hire, an organization must identify its goals for the training. These goals will guide the selection of content beyond the foundational topics described earlier. Hiring an MI trainer to work with rehabilitation groups can be difficult as many might not have experience working in this area of specialization. Two members of MINT, Carolina Yahne and Denise Ernst, published a list of 14 questions to ask MI trainers before hiring (MINT, 2021). Four of these questions are listed below as these will assist rehabilitation organizations in determining if the MI trainers are familiar with and able to customize the training appropriately:

1. Our audience will be composed of *rehabilitation professionals*. What experience do you have working with trainees such as ours, and what are some of the issues you see related to training our type of group?
2. Our trainees primarily work with patients/people with *newly acquired or chronic illnesses or injuries and disabilities*. What experience have you had with such issues?
3. In what ways can you tailor your training and materials for us? For example, can you train to a protocol that is already developed? Can you modify the materials to be focused on *rehabilitation*? How can you make the exercises relevant to our trainees?
4. If a trainee presented you with this kind of challenge, how would you handle it?

Measuring MI Training Effectiveness

When organizations invest resources and staff time for MI training as a quality improvement project or professional development program, it is imperative that the impact of the MI training program is measured. In fact, identifying outcomes and methods for measurement is a task that should happen early in the process. Sharing such outcomes can reinforce staff's dedication to MI and maintain enthusiasm over time. Most importantly, reporting these outcomes can justify training efforts and resources to organizational leadership. Organizations are unlikely to continue to devote precious resources to training programs that cannot prove return on investment.

To effectively measure the impacts of MI training, it is especially important that systems consider their desired impact in advance of training implementation and identify a few team members who will be able to devote time and resources to the evaluation of the training impact. Depending on the institution and desired outcomes, this may involve approval from an institutional review board, access to and ability to extract information from electronic medical records, and support for data collection and analysis. More information about MI training or intervention as a quality improvement project can be found in Chapter 13. This section will explore measurement constructs, specific outcomes, and methods of measurement.

LEARNER OUTCOMES

The impact of MI training on learners is an important set of outcomes to measure. If the MI training program cannot positively impact learners, then it will not impact patients or systems. Learner outcomes may differ based on the organization or institution but often include satisfaction with the training itself, knowledge and attitudes about MI, self-efficacy for using MI, frequency of use of MI skills, and quality of MI skills when used.

Satisfaction

Measuring learner satisfaction with MI training is typically done using a paper or online survey completed by learners immediately after training. Using an existing course satisfaction survey or one adapted from an organization's continuing education office can simplify the process. Such surveys should gather quantitative and qualitative data around general satisfaction with course content, accessibility and feasibility of the course, trainer materials, and training process. More specifically, the survey should gather data around applicability of course content to work roles, to what extent the learner's practice will change given the course content, and whether a learner would recommend the training to a colleague.

Knowledge and Attitudes

Learner knowledge and attitudes about MI is another construct that is likely to be impacted by MI training and therefore is commonly measured. For a practitioner to use MI skills effectively, they must first understand the fundamental principles and foundational spirit that underlie the MI skill set. The most frequently used tool to measure MI knowledge and attitudes is the Motivational Interviewing Knowledge and Attitudes Test (MIKAT; Leffingwell, 2006), which is specifically focused on understanding MI for patients with substance use and abuse conditions. The MIKAT, a true/false questionnaire, has been adapted for other patient populations, or to be more generalized in nature. This measure can be easily adapted for rehabilitation populations.

Self-Efficacy

Learners' beliefs and impressions about their ability to use MI can help us to understand the impact of MI training. This construct may be more specifically defined by factors like self-efficacy or confidence, sense of importance of using MI, and sense of feasibility of using MI. Self-efficacy, a construct considered and measured in many disciplines, can be conceptualized generally or more specifically. For the purposes of understanding the impact of MI training on learners, it is helpful to measure learners' sense of confidence in using MI specifically, rather than self-efficacy for their daily work. Similarly, measuring a learner's sense of how important MI is to their daily work and how realistic it will be for them to incorporate MI into their daily work will be more helpful than measuring generalized sense of importance and feasibility of their work.

A review of the literature shows that many self-efficacy questionnaires have been used in previous studies of MI training (e.g., Cucciare et al., 2012); however, to our knowledge, there is no standardized measure with published reliability and validity data in this context. One option is to use the MI rulers, commonly used to evaluate the impact of MI interventions with patient samples and found to have high reliability in this context (e.g., Boudreaux et al., 2012). Learners are asked to respond to the following three questions with a single numeric response on a scale of 0 (none) to 10 (completely). The questions used are often (a) Importance, "How important is it to you to use motivational interviewing skills in your work?"; (b) Confidence, "How confident are you that you can successfully incorporate motivational interviewing skills in your work?"; and (c) Feasibility, "How realistic is it for you to use motivational interviewing skills in your work?"

Larson and Martin (2021) recently published another measure called the Motivational Interviewing Confidence Survey, a 24-item self-report measure that invites practitioners to rate on a scale of 0 to 10 their confidence in demonstrating MI skills and principles. It was found to have good reliability. Examples of items from this measure include "On a scale of 0 to 10, how certain are you that you can solicit client participation despite recent client refusal?" and "On a scale of 0 to 10, how certain are you that you can provide affirmations to help the client identify strengths & past successes and support their motivation to change?" This measure addresses practitioner confidence with a level of detail that the MI rulers do not; however, it does not evaluate sense of importance or feasibility for using MI in work contexts.

Skills

The quality of learner MI skills and the frequency with which they are used are important outcomes to measure to determine the effectiveness of an MI training program as, of course, the goal of most training programs is to help practitioners evolve in MI skills so that they are more competent in using them in clinical contexts. The Helpful Responses Questionnaire (HRQ; Miller et al., 1991) was found to have high reliability and validity. The HRQ is a brief response questionnaire designed to measure therapeutic empathy and engagement-promoting communication skills. It involves six clinical vignettes to which the respondent writes "the next thing you would say" in response to the patient in that scenario. Responses are scored based on the presence and quality of foundational MI attitudes and skills. Given its length and its use of written responses, the HRQ is considered a less time-intensive and burdensome method for measuring MI skills. Since the HRQ is completed outside of clinical work, this measure does not calculate the frequency with which MI is being used.

The Video-Assessment of Simulated Encounters-Revised (VASE-R; Rosengren et al., 2008) is like the HRQ in that it asks the practitioner to write a response to a patient's statement that gets scored by a trained evaluator; however, the patient situation is presented via simulated video with patient actors rather than a written transcript. The VASE-R has been found to have reliability and validity levels that are similar to the HRQ. The challenge of using the VASE-R is having the equipment available to present the videos to the learners; this especially becomes a challenge when longitudinal measurement of MI skills is desired. Similar to the HRQ, the VASE-R does not measure the frequency of MI skill use.

The most time-intensive method for measuring learner MI skills is via a clinician behavioral sample that is either evaluated live by an MI expert or recorded via video and submitted to an MI expert for review. The MI expert then uses the MI Treatment Integrity (MITI 4; Moyers et al., 2016) system to score the interaction. This method can be considered burdensome as it requires the MI expert to have the time, ability, and permission to observe the practitioner with a patient, or it requires the practitioner to have the time, ability, and permission to record their interactions with a patient and submit to a third party. This method also requires that the MI expert is competent in using the MITI 4 coding system, which requires considerable formal training. This measurement tool does capture the frequency of MI skill use within a designated interaction or clinical encounter.

PATIENT OUTCOMES

Once it is demonstrated that an MI training improves the knowledge, attitudes, self-efficacy, and quality and frequency of MI skill use of a practitioner, it is valuable to demonstrate that those practitioner improvements are associated with improvements in identified patient outcomes. This is more likely to occur when the MI training is identified in the context of a quality improvement project, where a particular segment of clinical care is being targeted for change. For example, if a clinic identifies that patients are completing home exercise programs (HEPs) at low rates and wants to conduct MI training for therapists to improve their ability to communicate about HEPs, it would be reasonable to measure rate of HEP completion as a desired patient health outcome after training. Another example might be implementing MI training for rehabilitation nurses focused on increasing a patient's confidence in bowel management after spinal cord injury. In this case an appropriate patient health outcome to explore could be the number of times a patient independently performs their bowel program. Even without a specific MI training focus, it is possible that patient outcomes may be positively impacted; however, there will be many confounding factors to consider. Please review Chapter 13 to determine approaches for ensuring that these patient health outcomes are being measured and are accessible for analysis.

SYSTEM OUTCOMES

Many organizations that choose to implement MI training at the unit, clinic, or system level will be interested in measuring system-level outcomes such as readmission rates, show or no-show rates, and patient satisfaction with care or patient experience with care. Desired outcomes should align with the goals and mission of the institution.

Patient satisfaction or experience with care is a common system-level outcome that can be impacted by MI training of practitioners. That is, when rehabilitation practitioners become more skillful in MI, patients are more likely to experience a sense of partnership and collaboration in healthcare, which improves their perception of their quality of care. It can be challenging, however, to use total scores on standardized patient satisfaction or patient experience surveys to measure these impacts. Press Ganey surveys like the Hospital Consumer Assessment of Health Care Providers and Systems or the Clinician and Group Consumer Assessment of Health Care Providers and Systems assess many areas known to impact patient satisfaction with hospital and ambulatory healthcare services, including safety, environmental aesthetics, and accessibility. Therefore, subscales measuring the quality of provider–patient relationships, such as the Doctor Communication Subscale or the Nursing Communication Subscale, should be used.

In large organizations, partnering with a patient experience office or officer can be useful to identify the most appropriate system-level outcomes that are accessible and available for analysis. These prevents redoing work that has already been done or is being done. In smaller organizations, determining how a team or clinic is already measuring patient satisfaction with care (i.e., electronic survey delivered after each encounter), as an example, is an excellent place to start. When possible, capitalizing on measures that are already in use and therefore already built into workflows reduces burden on staff and patients alike.

Conclusion

MI is extremely helpful for practitioners working with patients and/or families who may be ambivalent about engaging in new health behaviors or health management strategies. This is extraordinarily relevant in the rehabilitation context. For some particularly motivated rehabilitation professionals, self-study of MI or self-selecting to participate in MI training will occur; however, most healthcare professionals believe that they do not need to improve their own communication skills or methodology. Therefore, rehabilitation practice or organization leadership may determine that MI training for all practitioners is an important best practice and will help achieve desired patient and system outcomes. Committing to MI training, including measuring outcomes and providing opportunities for sustaining MI skills, can help individuals, practices, and organizations achieve a culture of patient-centered care.

References

Agency for Healthcare Research and Quality. (2018). *The guide to improving patient safety in primary care settings by engaging patients and families.*

Agency for Healthcare Research and Quality. (n.d.). *CAHPS clinician & group survey.* Retrieved August 2021 from https://www.ahrq.gov/cahps/surveys-guidance/cg/index.html

Boudreaux, E. D., Sullivan, A., Abar, B., Bernstein, S. L., Ginde, A. A., & Camargo, C. A. (2012). Motivation rulers for smoking cessation: A prospective observational examination of construct and predictive validity. *Addiction Science and Clinical Practice, 7*, Article 8. https://doi.org/10.1186/1940-0640-7-8

Cucciare, M. A., Ketroser, N., Wilbourne, P., Midboe, A. M., Cronkite, R., Berg-Smith, S. M., & Chardos, J. (2012). Teaching motivational interviewing to primary care staff in the Veterans Health Administration. *Journal of General Internal Medicine, 27*(8), 953–961. https://doi.org/10.1007/s11606-012-2016-6

Helfrich, C. D., Li, Y. F., Sharp, N. D., & Sales, A. E. (2009). Organizational Readiness to Change Assessment (ORCA): Development of an instrument based on the Promoting Action on Research in Health Services (PARIHS) framework. *Implementation Science, 4*, Article 38. https://doi.org/10.1186/1748-5908-4-38

Knowles, M. S. (1984). *Andragogy in action.* Jossey-Bass.

Larson, E., & Martin, B. A. (2021). Measuring motivational interviewing self-efficacy of pre-service students completing a competency-based motivational interviewing course. *Exploratory Research in Clinical and Social Pharmacy, 1*, Article 100009. https://doi.org/10.1016/j.rcsop.2021.100009

Leffingwell, T. (2006). Motivational interviewing knowledge and attitudes test (MIKAT) for evaluation of training outcomes. *MINUET, 3*, 10–11.

Mezirow, J. (1991). *Transformative dimensions of adult learning.* Jossey-Bass.

Miller, W. R., & Rollnick, S. (1991). Motivational interviewing: Preparing people to change addictive behavior. The Guilford Press.

Miller, W. R., & Mount, K. A. (2001). A small study of training in motivational interviewing: Does one workshop change clinician and client behavior? *Behavioral and Cognitive Psychotherapy, 29*(4), 457–471. https://doi.org/10.1017/S1352465801004064

Motivational Interviewing Network of Trainers. (2021). *Training expectations.* https://motivationalinterviewing.org/training-expectations

Moyers, T. B., Rowell, L. N., Manuel, J. K., Ernst, D., & Houck, J. M. (2016). The Motivational Interviewing Treatment Integrity Code (MITI 4): Rationale, preliminary reliability and validity. *Journal of Substance Abuse Treatment, 65*, 36–42. https://doi.org/10.1016/j.jsat.2016.01.001

Rosengren, D. B., Hartzler, B., Baer, J. S., Wells, E. A., & Dunn, C. W. (2008). The Video Assessment of Simulated Encounters—Revised (VASE-R): Reliability and validity of a revised measure of motivational interviewing skills. *Drug and Alcohol Dependence, 97*(1–2), 130–138. https://doi.org/10.1016/j.drugalcdep.2008.03.018

Schwalbe, C. S., Oh, H. Y., & Zweben, A. (2014). Sustaining motivational interviewing: A meta-analysis of training studies. *Addiction, 109*(8), 1287–1294. https://doi.org/10.1111/add.12558

Shea, C. M., Jacobs, S. R., Esserman, D. A., Bruce, K., & Weiner, B. J. (2014). Organizational readiness for implementing change: A psychometric assessment of a new measure. *Implementation Science, 9*, Article 7. https://doi.org/10.1186/1748-5908-9-7

Soderlund, L. L., Madson, M. B., Rubak, S., & Nilsen, P. (2011). A systemic review of motivational interviewing training for general health care practitioners. *Patient Education and Counseling, 84*(1), 16–26.

Thomson, R., Fichten, C. S., Havel, A., Budd, J., & Asuncion, J. (2015). Blending universal design, e-learning, and information and communication technologies. In S. E. Burgstahler (Ed.), *Universal design in higher education: From principles to practice* (2nd ed., pp. 275–284). Harvard Education Press.

13 Motivational Interviewing and Quality Improvement Research

Amanda Choflet, Annette Lavezza, and Kelly Daley

Introduction

In the years since it was first described as a novel approach in 1980, motivational interviewing (MI) spirit and skills have been successfully implemented with positive findings in diverse clinical settings, including numerous chronic diseases (cardiovascular care, diabetes, rehabilitation; Aubeeluck et al., 2021; Dehghan-Nayeri et al., 2019; Jamil et al., 2021). First developed as a new therapeutic approach in patients with substance use disorders, MI represented a clinical innovation that was described in theoretical terms and subsequently tested prospectively with increasingly diverse patient populations (Miller & Rose, 2009). In other words, MI began organically in clinical practice, was described by researchers and tested in research studies, then was adapted to novel clinical environments in both implementation studies as well as quality improvement (QI) projects.

While a number of studies have reported both positive and null findings with the utilization of MI in clinical settings, some compelling patterns have begun to emerge, such as improved efficacy in traditionally underserved populations and in some clinician groups over others (Gaume et al, 2016; Miller & Rose, 2009). Even with numerous studies indicating the usefulness of MI in various settings, a debate

Amanda Choflet, Annette Lavezza, and Kelly Daley, *Motivational Interviewing and Quality Improvement Research* In: *Motivational Interviewing in Medical Rehabilitation*. Edited by: Nicole Schechter, Connie Jacocks, Lester Butt, and Stephen T. Wegener, Oxford University Press. © Oxford University Press 2024. DOI: 10.1093/oso/9780197748268.003.0014 is underway regarding the most efficacious settings, diseases, and clinician teams in which to initiate MI practices.

Despite its usefulness in a variety of patient care settings and situations, it is sometimes difficult to understand or articulate the distinct value of MI approaches to patient care. This is further complicated by the finding that MI may be especially useful when combined with additional active treatments, making it even more difficult to find causal relationships between MI programs and patient outcomes (Miller & Rose, 2009). Structured, systematic QI strategies, coupled with clinical research based on implementation science principles can be applied to broaden the understanding of MI in the clinical setting. This chapter will outline a variety of approaches to systematically measuring the impact of MI spirit and skills on clinical care, focusing not only on QI techniques but also on research opportunities and the utilization of implementation science frameworks.

How Does MI Work Anyway?

In order to produce evidence regarding the effectiveness of MI, it is necessary to understand the theoretical framework driving MI as an intervention strategy. With patient/client behavior change being the ultimate goal, it is assumed that a relationship exists between (1) clinician–patient interaction, (2) patient change talk and commitment to behavior change, and (3) actual behavior change. In other words, MI-consistent behavior by the clinician should lead to change talk by the patient, which then leads to behavior change, a process that has been demonstrated in actual clinical settings (Romano et al., 2017). Given these assumptions, evaluation opportunities exist at each point in the framework, from clinician training (post-training evaluations, observations using standardized patients, etc.) to the clinician–patient interaction (documenting MI dose, screening results, etc.) to patient response to the interaction (documenting patient change talk and commitment to change using readiness rulers, self-assessment techniques, etc.) to actual behavior change (documenting actual behaviors and patient outcomes).

Another way to think about the process of MI is to consider the MI spirit, which involves the principles of acceptance, collaboration, empowerment, and compassion (Mullen et al., 2020) as well as the MI skills necessary to achieve the desired outcome, which may include things like using open-ended questions, affirmations, reflective listening, and summarizing (Miller & Rollnick, 2013; Miller & Rollnick, 2023). Please refer to Chapters 1 and 3, respectively, for a more in-depth review of MI spirit and MI skills. Effective MI will include both relational and directional components requiring both MI spirit and skills (Morgenstern et al., 2017), and therefore, both components must be measured and documented in order to produce robust evaluation results.

MEASURING THE MI "DOSE" AND FIDELITY

Regardless of the type of MI program being implemented (research, QI, or implementation science), it is critical that the "dosage" of MI is measured as accurately as possible. This dosage must include elements of both the spirit, or relational component, and skills, or technical component, of the MI intervention. While the gold standard of ensuring fidelity to MI principles and skills is direct observation by a peer evaluator, this approach is not realistic in many clinical settings. If a team lacks the resources or time to implement peer observation, an alternative approach to measurement is recommended, such as role playing, simulations using standardized patients, or pre- and post-tests in conjunction with training sessions. If possible, it is important to track the behaviors and attitudes of the clinician as well as the specific MI skills being utilized and the specific health promotion topics being addressed. Quantifiable metrics are most helpful when justifying future resource allocation to support MI efforts. Please refer to Chapter 12 for more in-depth information regarding MI training and training resources.

QI

Because the evidence supporting MI in a variety of clinical settings is so robust, many clinical environments will begin their work with MI by developing a QI project that incorporates MI principles and skills. QI is defined as the framework used to "systematically improve the ways that patient care is delivered" (Agency for Healthcare Research and Quality, 2013). QI often begins by identifying a problem within a system and implementing strategies to address it (Bauer et al., 2015). Change often occurs based on small changes where a goal is set, a change is made, outcomes are assessed, and modifications are implemented (Arbuckle et al., 2020). Often, this process follows a formal cycle such as the plan–do–study–act cycle. This cycle is often considered a rapid cycle of change addressing small-scale changes before broader adoption occurs (McQuillan et al., 2016). Current practice is measured, best practices are identified and implemented, changes are measured and evaluated, then the cycle begins anew. Importantly, this process is designed to improve clinical outcomes in as close to real time as possible, without necessarily generating new knowledge or rigorously measuring the outcomes of the improvement process itself. QI is a very useful approach when working with a population, disease, and setting in which MI has been shown to be effective and the clinical team is attempting to improve internal clinical practice and patient outcomes as quickly and efficiently as possible.

Research

Research is required when best practices are not clearly defined for a clinical environment or population and new knowledge must be discovered. The history of MI as a specific clinical approach with a later-appearing theory helps one to understand the symbiotic relationship between clinical practice and research. MI research has been particularly concerned with validating and testing the "secret sauce" of the clinician–patient interaction and relationship in inducing positive patient outcomes. There is still much room for clarity around the interaction of the MI spirit and skills in evoking patient readiness for change and subsequent behavior change.

MI research can focus on any aspect or application of MI, from clinician training to participant interaction to patient outcomes. Much of the research regarding MI has necessarily focused on the clinician's skills and spirit in delivering effective MI interventions in specific clinical settings. Because the hypothesized action of MI involves skills that are observable from a quantitative and a qualitative perspective, MI research may benefit from a mixed-methods approach that incorporates both quantitative and qualitative data. Some researchers have attempted to isolate and articulate specific MI-consistent actions on the part of the clinician that may be measured as part of an MI research or QI project. These measures would be considered *process metrics*, while the patient outcomes that resulted from these clinician behaviors would be considered *patient outcomes metrics*.

The gold standard of MI research is to directly observe clinician and patient interactions in order to assess MI-consistent spirit and skills. This has made MI research a fairly expensive undertaking since measuring MI skills requires either that clinicians must be observed while delivering patient care or that workflows and evaluation tools are in place to measure MI dose, patient response and readiness, and patient outcomes in real time. Adding to the complexity, MI spirit and skills are not static but rather are responsive and adaptive, sometimes resulting in messy data points with unclear results. Some researchers have begun deploying technological solutions such as natural language processing to code clinician–patient interactions (Tanana et al., 2016), but this only reduces one time-intensive component of MI research.

Another barrier to MI research is the length of time needed to study patient outcomes from the initiation of MI intervention. With MI, patient outcomes may need to be tracked over a long period of time before findings can be concluded.

Implementation Science

Implementation science involves the systematic application of best practices in a new clinical environment with structured evaluation metrics. Defined by Eccles and Mittman (2006) as "the scientific study of methods to promote the systematic uptake of research findings and other evidence-based practices into routine practice," this approach strives to address challenges with integrating new research results in a timely fashion given that past performance indicates that it can take up to 17 years to integrate new evidence into practice (Bauer et al., 2015).

Implementation science focuses on approaches to support the integration of new knowledge. There are frameworks to support this approach. One such framework, seen in Figure 13.1, the translating research into practice (TRiP) model, is a specific method that supports systemic integration of research (Pronovost et al., 2008). The model consists of four steps: summarizing the evidence, identifying barriers, measuring performance, and ensuring that all patients receive the intervention.

Prior to starting model steps, the team should identify and engage key stakeholders who will be impacted by the approach. In addition, success is influenced by the core team. Core teams in rehabilitation often include multiple disciplines (e.g., physical therapy, occupational therapy [OT], nursing), all of which can benefit from MI, so all disciplines should be engaged at the very beginning of the process.

Since TRiP is focused on implementing current evidence, during the first step of summarizing the evidence, it is important to review intervention options and strategically select options with the best expected outcomes and fewest barriers. Once the evidence is summarized, the core team should review the proposed implementation

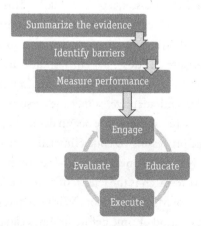

FIGURE 13.1 Translating Evidence Into Practice (TriP) Model

plan in detail to identify possible barriers; this might include walking through the process with each discipline and assessing the challenges.

The next key component in TRiP is to measure performance. Strategic decisions about measurement should be made at this point in the process. Clinical care, and specifically rehabilitation, can and must produce primary measurements of clinical performance. These measurement data are often from the documentation in the electronic health record (EHR). While the EHR produces large data sets, it often needs specific enhancements in order to systematically collect indicators of compliance with MI interventions, assessments, or outcomes. Therefore, when assessing whether the EHR information is sufficient, one may examine specifics in EHR collection of standardized MI clinician interventions. If enhancements are necessary, it will be vital to build partnerships with those who have internal knowledge and ability to build in the EHR, mine necessary data, and create informative reports.

The final step in TRiP is ensuring that all patients receive the intervention. This component requires engaging, educating, executing, and evaluating (*4 Es*) at the front lines. First, front-line providers are engaged in the change by providing evidence and rationale for the change and details about the intervention. Next, the providers are educated on the intervention. The core team might then develop tools to execute. Finally, front-line providers are given feedback on performance and metrics to evaluate performance.

CHOOSING AN APPROACH

Whether choosing to use a QI or implementation science approach, there are key items to consider. Most importantly, identify whether the team is initially implementing MI or refining an MI intervention. If the team is beginning the journey and there is an identified need for systemic culture change, perhaps selecting an implementation science approach would be more beneficial. If the team has already adopted components but needs to refine MI implementation, perhaps a QI approach that yields rapid change would be appropriate.

Regardless of the approach selected, the ability to measure success and provide feedback to the team is crucial. It will be imperative to define measurement before starting the project. Determining precise measures of study is a highly specific step the core team must take to ensure that these measures can exist efficiently and accurately in the recording clinicians' EHR workflow. For example, if an OT is to indicate that MI was utilized during a session,

1. Is there a check box in the documentation view indicating this fidelity to the intervention (numerator for compliance of the process)?

2. Does there need to be more detail recorded about the nature of the MI intervention and the client's response, and if so, where will this be done in the EHR?

3. If it does not already exist, is this supported by the literature and copyright-approved for the EHR?

4. For the EHR workflow, can the clinician record this information efficiently without leaving their usual EHR documentation view?

5. Looking at the bigger picture, are there indicators that this patient was appropriate for MI to begin with (denominator for compliance)?

Measurement and Evaluation

The measurement of clinical outcomes with the use of MI techniques is critical for a number of reasons. Without outcomes-oriented implementation strategies, MI techniques are obfuscated by traditional practice approaches. It has been well established that MI approaches may cost more money in the short term but may lead to better long-term patient outcomes (Dwommoh et al., 2018). Because of the relatively higher cost of MI approaches to patient care, it is critical to develop outcome measurements that create an understanding of the "value proposition" that moves beyond the traditional short-term fiscal and QI cycle. More important than choosing the "perfect" measurements for an MI project is choosing metrics that match the maturity of the MI project itself. The team must systematically determine which data are already being collected and develop an implementation plan that builds from current processes.

MI skills may be particularly difficult to measure not only because they are difficult to isolate from more task-focused clinical care but also because the outcomes may not be immediately apparent or measurable. Overall, there are two primary types of outcome measurements. The first is process outcomes, which are those metrics concerned with the processes involved with bringing new skills or practices into care. The second is patient outcomes, which measure the actual clinical outcomes in the patient or patient population being targeted. Patient outcomes can be measured using quantitative, qualitative, or mixed-methods approaches. Examples of each type of measurement are shown in Table 13.1.

There are many reasons for choosing specific process and patient outcome measurements, and the most holistic approach utilizes both types of metrics. Process outcomes are more closely associated with QI and implementation frameworks, though they can be important considerations with original research as well. Patient

TABLE 13.1

Examples of Process and Outcome Measurement of Motivational Interviewing

	Process	Patient outcomes
Short term	• Team training (complete/ incomplete; pre-/post-training evaluations) • Uptake of MI skills by team members via direct observation • Quality of the MI skills being used • Documented referrals to substance use treatment, other services • Documented delivery of MI dose itself (time, tools utilized, number of conversations, topics discussed)	• Decreased reported substance use (AUDIT-C, DAST, etc.) • Functional outcomes • Emotional outcomes (PHQ, GAD, etc.) • QOL outcomes (HRQOL) • Physical activity levels • Patient journals (qualitative analysis) • Disease-related outcomes (acute)
Middle and long term	• Program satisfaction • Participant adherence/ engagement	• Functional outcomes • Disease-related outcomes (long-term, chronic) • Work-related outcomes • Return to work (Aanesen, 2020) • Sickness-related absences (Aasdahl, 2018)

Note: AUDIT-C = Alcohol Use Disorders Identification Test—Concise; DAST = Drug Abuse Screening Test; GAD = Generalized Anxiety Disorder Assessment; HRQOL = health-related quality of life; MI = motivational interviewing; PHQ = Patient Health Questionnaire; QOL = quality of life.

outcomes are important in all approaches. The relative benefits and drawbacks of each type of outcome measurement are described in Table 13.2.

Tracking specific process improvement and patient care outcomes will lead to a better understanding of clinical approaches and both the short- and long-term impacts of utilizing MI skills. In all measurement approaches, it is critical to describe and measure the MI skills, techniques, frequency, and duration of the MI intervention received by the patient.

TABLE 13.2

Benefits and Drawbacks of Outcome Measurements

	Process	Patient outcomes
Benefits	• More amenable to EHR functionality • Shorter-term measurements • Less costly to measure • More objective	• Longer-range measurement period • More amenable to narrative/qualitative • Potential for more meaningful patient results
Drawbacks	• Does not usually measure actual patient outcomes (less likely to justify continued support for the program or generate new knowledge)	• More reliant on specialized forms or documentation requirements (current EHR build may not capture most important/relevant patient outcomes) • Usually costlier to measure • More subjective

Note: EHR = electronic health record.

Putting the EHR to Work

It is often a significant challenge to collect embedded measures of process and patient outcomes (Daley, 2018). Access to data to create implementation-supportive reporting can be a barrier for many organizations (Van Wert et al., 2021). A useful approach is to begin with the final reports needed in mind, which must show patient outcomes and the processes that supported them. The study team will need to spend time with these detailed considerations (Daley et al., 2020). In fact, creating mock-ups of these needed reports will serve teams well. For example, in order to perform the *execute* step of TRiP, leadership will need to specify in detail what is needed in order to provide feedback to the core team about the intervention compliance rate. This rate is described as the count of times the intervention is provided (numerator) over the count of times when it should have been provided (denominator). Frequent reports in team huddles show trends in uptake of the implementation in summary form, such as in Table 13.3, and in detailed form by clinician and by client in order to understand and resolve challenges in data collection.

Data from the reports will also need to be utilized for scientific analysis. The report design should make clear to what extent clients receiving MI are achieving a certain threshold for improvement in outcome. This is frequently calculated as the

TABLE 13.3

Electronic Health Record Considerations—Example of Summary Report of Compliance to Intervention

Month	Visits with opportunity to provide MI	Visits with MI intervention completed (Compliant)	Compliance rate
Jan	27	17	63.0%
Feb	40	25	62.5%
Mar	44	25	56.8%
Apr	39	24	61.5%
May	31	24	77.4%

Note: MI = motivational interviewing.

amount of change in outcome measure over time but can become much more complex when considering ceiling effects and the stratification of patients based upon age, comorbidities, etc.

It may be found that there is a gap in the information being collected in the EHR. Perhaps the data gap was found in the initial assessment of data needs. Perhaps a change occurred in the EHR build that requires attention, or the data point does not exist for a subset of those involved in documenting the implementation. This assessment can be guided by the questions listed in Table 13.4.

Teams are likely to need to request to build specific data entry into the EHR. Once you determine to whom and what form you must make this request, there are a few additional things to keep in mind which can enhance your chances for success:

1. Make the request as easy as possible to understand and build.
   a. Use screen shots of the current EHR with arrows to show exactly where you propose the new documentation be located.
   b. Mock up what the new entry will look like including selection lists using standard office software (i.e., Word or Excel).
   c. Spell out everything; do not use abbreviations.

2. In order to advocate for build priority, include information clearly linking it to organizational initiatives if at all possible. Spend some time finding organizational, clinical, or operational champions to help support its linkage to important initiatives. You may consider linking your build to:
   a. quality care
   b. patient safety
   c. reduction in unplanned 30-day readmissions

TABLE 13.4

Electronic Health Record Considerations for Quality Improvement, Implementation Science, or Research

Question to ask	Examples of EHR data or processes
Do all required measures of fidelity to intervention (process) exist in EHR? (Numerator for use of specific intervention/ denominator for count of times when intervention should be used)	Indicator of clinician MI spirit Measure of dose/frequency and/or duration Clinician assessment of how well MI skills were utilized (e.g., *very strong, strong, weak, very weak*)
Do all required measures of client response to intervention exist in EHR?	Indicator of diminished resistance, commitment to identified behavior change
Do all required measures of client health outcome exist in the EHR?	Behavior change; PHQ score, HRQOL score; physical activity levels (distance walked journal, AM-PAC)
Do all required related data points exist in EHR? (Client demographics, comorbidities, referral information, visit information, clinician identifiers)	Number of qualifying visits, visit dates, patient age, patient gender, clinician ID
Is collection in the EHR in a "discrete" and reportable fashion versus "free text"?	PHQ-9 raw score (0–27) numeric database storage
Is collection efficient to document and in the clinician's usual workflow (i.e., not required to go "find" the place to enter information)?	End user login to view points of entry by each clinician type
Is there no confusion about where/how to document in the EHR/not redundant?	Work with end users to view all points of entry of same information
Which data points do not exist in the EHR but could be collected via another method? And how to merge with study database?	Numbers and names of clinicians in a department (from staff roster), long-term outcome (e.g., from follow-up phone call), training and competency dates
Can the project/study be conducted without all data points on the "wish list"?	Focus and refocus upon minimum data set and feasibility of systematic collection
Must you request and advocate with the organizational EHR committee/ stakeholders to add or edit current data point entry?	Knowledge of the people and organizational structure for EHR enhancements
Must you request data reporting for core team feedback or scientific inquiry?	Knowledge of the people and structure for reporting requests and data governance

Note: AM-PAC = Activity Measure for Post Acute Care; EHR = electronic health record; HRQOL = health-related quality of life; MI = motivational interviewing; PHQ = Patient Health Questionnaire (PHQ-9 = nine-item PHQ).

    d. documentation efficiency

    e. length of stay

    f. number of visits/cost

    g. client satisfaction

3. Seek to understand and leverage how EHR enhancement work is prioritized and assigned to a builder.

4. When the builder has questions, respond swiftly and very concretely with
as little jargon as possible.

Case Study

QI IMPLEMENTATION OF A SCREENING, BRIEF INTERVENTION, AND
REFERRAL TO TREATMENT PROGRAM IN A REHABILITATION SETTING

Reagan worked with traumatic brain injury (TBI) patients in the outpatient rehabilitation clinic in an urban academic hospital on the east coast of the United States. After
several of her patients reported substance use issues while engaged in rehabilitation,
she became concerned that the rehabilitation clinic was not doing enough to help TBI
patients with risky alcohol and drug use. She was especially affected by the death of
one patient, who successfully completed rehabilitation for their TBI and subsequently
died from an accidental drug overdose. The doctors, nurses, and social workers were
doing everything they knew to do for patients with known alcohol and drug-related
problems but commented frequently that they felt unprepared to give helpful advice
to their patients and that they were "in the dark" about providing real resources.

Reagan determined key stakeholders interested in addressing the issue and con-
vened a small core team of doctors, nurses, social workers, clinical nurse specialists, and advanced practice providers to develop an action plan to better support
these patients. The team chose to follow the TRiP model to translate evidence into
practice.

The first step of the model is to summarize the evidence. The core team reviewed
literature from primary care, emergency medicine, and rehabilitation medicine.
Results of the literature review revealed basic practices for prescribing opioid medications, routine drug testing, and use of validated screening tools for substance abuse
potential. They then began Phase 2 of TRiP by considering local barriers to implementation of the previously identified interventions. For example, Reagan knew
that asking rehabilitation physicians and nurses to use a long, unfamiliar screening
tool in routine practice was unrealistic, especially without a plan for what to do once
positive screens were identified.

The measure performance phase of the TRiP model was initiated when the team consulted the substance use literature again to learn more about screening tools and intervention options in the case of positive screens. Through this search, the core team identified the screening, brief intervention, and referral to treatment (SBIRT) approach program recommended by the Substance Abuse and Mental Health Services Administration. The team selected SBIRT because it was shown to be effective in reducing risky alcohol consumption in primary care and emergency room settings, which are considered similar to rehabilitation settings. The core team reviewed several public health–oriented resources to guide the implementation of SBIRT.

At this point, the team identified an additional local barrier. The team lacked training on the brief intervention part of SBIRT, and they did not have anyone on their staff who could conduct such training. Therefore, the team returned to Step 1 of the TRiP process by reviewing the literature to determine appropriate methods for receiving training in SBIRT. As a result, the team was able to identify a faculty member within their system who was expertly trained in SBIRT and competent in delivering training to the rehabilitation team.

Once SBIRT was selected as the intervention, the team needed to address details related to measuring performance. The desired screening tool was not available in the department's existing documentation in EHR. Thus, collaboration with EHR partners to build the tool was required. The team worked with the EHR partner to develop an electronic documentation infrastructure using validated instruments for SBIRT and clinical decision support in patients' EHR. They incorporated validated instruments for screening (the Alcohol Use Disorders Identification Test—Concise [AUDIT-C]) and a single-question drug screen. These forms allowed data to populate patients' medical records and enter the data system, which facilitated retrospective, aggregate data collection. The forms included a clinical decision support feature that automatically totaled results from screenings and assessments. The introduction of the changes to the EHR ensured that all providers would have access to the screening and intervention.

In order to measure successful integration of MI approaches, the team selected a pre- and post-training assessment of team members' brief intervention skills, knowledge, and self-efficacy. They completed a baseline assessment of these three outcomes for all team members. In addition, the team piloted SBIRT from start to finish, including the use of the EHR forms with embedded screening tools, to establish a clinic baseline.

With the measures selected and baseline measured, the core team moved on to implement the intervention, using the 4 Es as a guide: engaging, educating, executing, and evaluating. This iterative process began with engaging, by which the team leaders held meetings with front-line staff to provide the rationale and purpose of the new SBIRT intervention. For education, the SBIRT trainer provided workshops to all rehabilitation team members so that they could build their own skills, knowledge, and self-efficacy for delivering SBIRT to patients.

To execute, the team developed an electronic toolkit for bedside clinicians so that they could quickly pull up a guide for completing SBIRT when a patient screened positive for risky substance use. The toolkits were installed on the clinic intranet and contained resources for low-, moderate-, and high-risk patients to simplify the process for clinicians. The evaluation phase involved a 3-month tracking period of the clinic's screening rates. As a result, the team discovered inconsistent use of the AUDIT screening tool. As such, the team decided to switch to a shorter but still validated screening tool. This cycle of continuous assessment, modification, and implementation allowed the team to continue to make improvements in performance over time.

Conclusion

QI is an extraordinarily valuable method that leads to important changes, which can improve the quality of care patients receive and, ultimately, patient health outcomes. When identifying MI as an intervention to include as part of a QI project, it is critical to have a foundation of a strong team with trusting relationships and a willingness to engage in flexible and strategic planning. Implementing MI as an intervention in and of itself or as part of a larger intervention requires commitment to a process of structured performance improvement and research, which is typically more important than the individual project at hand.

References

Aanesen, F., Berg, R., Løchting, I., Tingulstad, A., Eik, H., Storheim, K., Grotle, M., & Øiestad, B. E. (2021). Motivational interviewing and return to work for people with musculoskeletal disorders: A systematic mapping review. *Journal of Occupational Rehabilitation, 31*(1), 63–71. https://doi.org/10.1007/s10926-020-09892-0

Aasdahl, L., Pape, K., Vasseljen, O., Johnsen, R., Gismervik, S., Halsteinli, V., Fleten, N., Nielsen, C. V., & Fimland, M. S. (2018). Effect of inpatient multicomponent occupational rehabilitation versus less comprehensive outpatient rehabilitation on sickness absence in persons with musculoskeletal- or mental Health Disorders: A randomized clinical trial. *Journal of occupational rehabilitation, 28*(1), 170–179. https://doi.org/10.1007/s10926-017-9708-z

Agency for Healthcare Research and Quality. (2013). *Module 4. Approaches to quality improvement.* Retrieved June 20, 2021, from https://www.ahrq.gov/sites/default/files/wysiwyg/

cahps/quality-improvement/improvement-guide/4-approach-qi-process/cahps-section-4-ways-to-approach-qi-process.pdf

Arbuckle, M. R., Foster, F. P., Talley, R. M., Covell, N. H., & Essock, S. M. (2020). Applying motivational interviewing strategies to enhance organizational readiness and facilitate implementation efforts. *Quality Management in Health Care, 29*(1), 1–6. https://doi.org/10.1097/QMH.0000000000000234

Aubeeluck, E., Al-Arkee, S., Finlay, K., & Jalal, Z. (2021). The impact of pharmacy care and motivational interviewing on improving medication adherence in patients with cardiovascular diseases: A systematic review of randomised controlled trials. *International Journal of Clinical Practice, 75*(11), Article e14457. https://doi.org/10.1111/ijcp.14457

Bauer, M. S., Damschroder, L., Hagedorn, H., Smith, J., & Kilbourne, A. M. (2015). An introduction to implementation science for the non-specialist. *BMC Psychology, 3*, Article 32. https://doi.org/10.1186/s40359-015-0089-9

Daley, K. (2018). Adding power to systems science in rehabilitation. *Physical Therapy, 98*(8), 725–726. https://doi.org/10.1093/ptj/pzy061

Daley, K., Krushel, D., & Chevan, J. (2020). The physical therapist informatician as an enabler of capacity in a data-driven environment: An administrative case report. *Physiotherapy Theory and Practice, 36*(10), 1153–1163. https://doi.org/10.1080/09593985.2018.1548045

Dehghan-Nayeri, N., Ghaffari, F., Sadeghi, T., & Mozaffari, N. (2019). Effects of motivational interviewing on adherence to treatment regimens among patients with type 1 diabetes: A systematic review. *Diabetes Spectrum, 32*(2), 112–117. https://doi.org/10.2337/ds18-0038

Dwommoh, R., Sorsdahl, K., Myers, B., Asante, K. P., Naledi, T., Stein, D. J., & Cleary, S. (2018). Brief interventions to address substance use among patients presenting to emergency departments in resource poor settings: A cost-effectiveness analysis. *Cost Effectiveness and Resource Allocation, 16*, Article 24. https://doi.org/10.1186/s12962-018-0109-8

Eccles, M. P., & Mittman, B. S. (2006). Welcome to *Implementation Science*. *Implementation Science, 1*(1), Article 1. https://doi.org/10.1186/1748-5908-1-1

Gaume, J., Longabaugh, R., Magill, M., Bertholet, N., Gmel, G., & Daeppen, J. (2016). Under what conditions? Therapist and client characteristics moderate the role of change talk in brief motivational intervention. *Journal of Consulting and Clinical Psychology, 84*(3), 211–220. https://doi.org/10.1037/a0039918

Jamil, A., Javed, A., & Iqbal, M. (2021). Effects of motivational interviewing with conventional physical therapy on rehabilitation of chronic musculoskeletal disorders: A quasi-experimental study. *Journal of Pakistan Medical Association, 71*(4), 1123–1127. https://doi.org/10.47391/JPMA.873

McQuillan, R. F., Silver, S. A., Harel, Z., Weizman, A., Thomas, A., Bell, C., Chertow, G. M., Chan, C. T., & Nesrallah, G. (2016). How to measure and interpret quality improvement data. *Clinical Journal of the American Society of Nephrology, 11*(5), 908–914. https://doi.org/10.2215/CJN.11511015

Miller, W., & Rose, G. (2009). Toward a theory of motivational interviewing. *American Psychology, 64*(6), 527–537. https://doi.org/10.1037/a0016830

Miller, W., & Rollnick, S. (2013). *Motivational interviewing: Helping people change* (3rd ed.). Guilford Press.

Miller, W., & Rollnick, S. (2023). *Motivational interviewing: Helping people change and grow.* Guilford Press.

Morgenstern, J., Kuerbis, A., Houser, J., Levak, S., Amrhein, P., Shao, S., & McKay, J. (2017). Dismantling motivational interviewing: Effects on initiation of behavior change among problem drinkers seeking treatment. *Psychology of Addictive Behaviors, 31*(7), 751–762. https://doi. org/10.1037/adb0000317

Mullen, A., Isobel, S., Flanagan, K., Key, K., Dunbar, A., Bell, A., & Lewin, T. (2020). Motivational interviewing: Reconciling recovery-focused care and mental health nursing practice. *Issues in Mental Health Nursing, 41*(9), 807–814. https://doi.org/10.1080/01612840.2020.1731891

Pronovost, P. J., Berenholtz, S. M., & Needham, D. M. (2008). Translating evidence into practice: A model for large scale knowledge translation. *The BMJ, 337*, Article a1714. https://doi. org/10.1136/bmj.a1714

Romano, M., Arambasic, J., & Peters, L. (2017). Therapist and client interactions in motivational interviewing for social anxiety disorder. *Journal of Clinical Psychology, 73*(7), 829–847. https:// doi.org/10.1002/jclp.22405

Tanana, M., Hallgren, K., Imel, Z., Atkins, D., & Srikumar, V. (2016). A comparison of natural language processing methods for automated coding of motivational interviewing. *Journal of Substance Abuse Treatment, 65*, 43–50. https://doi.org/10.1016/j.jsat.2016.01.006

Van Wert, M. J., Malik, M., Memel, B., Moore, R., Buccino, D., Hackerman, F., Kumari, S., Everett, A., & Narrow, W. (2021). Provider perceived barriers and facilitators to integrating routine outcome monitoring into practice in an urban community psychiatry clinic: A mixed-methods quality improvement project. *Journal of Evaluation in Clinical Practice, 27*(4), 767–775. https://doi.org/10.1111/jep.13457

Index